Effective Strategies for Integrating

Social-Emotional Learning

in Your

Classroom

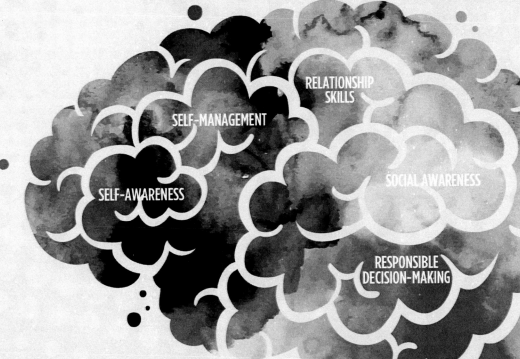

RELATIONSHIP SKILLS

SELF-MANAGEMENT

SELF-AWARENESS

SOCIAL AWARENESS

RESPONSIBLE DECISION-MAKING

ERICK J. HERRMANN, M.A.T.

Publishing Credits

Corinne Burton, M.A.Ed., *Publisher*
Aubrie Nielsen, M.S.Ed., *EVP of Content Development*
Véronique Bos, *Creative Director*
Cathy Hernandez, *Senior Content Manager*
Sara Johnson, M.S.Ed., *Editor*
Laureen Gleason, *Editor*
David Slayton, *Assistant Editor*

Image Credits

All images from iStock and/or Shutterstock

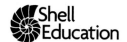

A division of Teacher Created Materials
5482 Argosy Avenue
Huntington Beach, CA 92649-1039
www.tcmpub.com/shell-education
ISBN 978-1-0876-4885-9
© 2022 Shell Educational Publishing, Inc.

Table of Contents

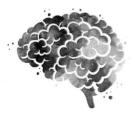

Preface 7

Introduction 11

   Why Social-Emotional Learning? 11

   School + SEL = Success 12

   Defining Social-Emotional Learning 14

   Social-Emotional Learning and the Standards 20

   SEL, Social Justice, and Equity 23

   Instruction and Social-Emotional Learning 24

   Stop and Reflect 27

Chapter 1: Self-Awareness 29

   Defining Self-Awareness 29

   Building a Sense of Self 32

   Identifying Personality Traits and Character Strengths 36

   Identifying and Naming Feelings 39

   Using Self-Reflection as a Tool 44

   Reflecting on Uncomfortable Feelings 50

   Building Students' Mindfulness 53

   Using Metacognition as a Tool 57

   Stop and Reflect 65

Chapter 2: Self-Management 67

   Defining Self-Management 67

   The Importance of Self-Management 68

   Teaching Self-Management Skills 69

   Proactive Strategies 70

   Cognitive Strategies 72

   Impulse Control 73

   Self-Talk 75

Self-Regulation. 77

Stop and Reflect. 85

Chapter 3: Social Awareness 87

Defining Social Awareness 87

The Role of Emotions. 87

The Role of Social Cues 94

Active Listening 96

The Reflective Cycle 104

The Role of Social Justice 105

Empathy as a Key Social-Awareness Skill 107

Stop and Reflect. 115

Chapter 4: Relationship Skills. 117

Defining Relationship Skills. 117

Modeling Positive Relationship Skills. 120

Systems for Building Relationships. 121

Team-Building Activities 127

Collaborative Learning to Build Relationships 131

Communication Skills to Build Relationships 134

Kindness and Gratitude: Key Relationship Skills 138

Relationship Management through Conflict Resolution. 140

Tips for Maintaining Relationships 141

Stop and Reflect. 143

Chapter 5: Responsible Decision-Making 145

Defining Responsible Decision-Making. 145

The Decision for Social Justice 146

Teaching Responsible Decision-Making. 147

The Decision-Making Process. 149

Developing Student Autonomy 151

Decision-Making in Action 160

Stop and Reflect. 167

Chapter 6: Putting It All Together. 169

How to Start 169

Into, Through, and Beyond: An SEL Framework for Success 171

The WOOP Strategy 174

School-Wide Implementation of SEL. 178

Addressing Self-Care 181

Final Thoughts. 182

Stop and Reflect. 183

References Cited. 185

Digital Resources 191

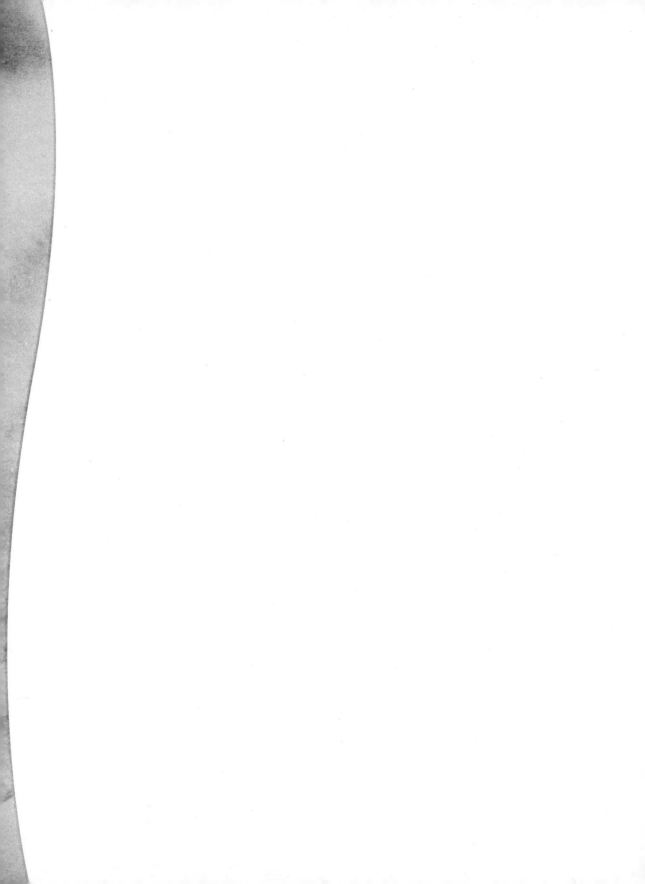

Preface

When I was growing up, my family did not discuss feelings in great depth. Don't get me wrong; I come from a loving family where we care deeply about one another. We just did not, and for the most part still do not, have a family culture where we discuss our feelings in great depth. My wife Natalie's family, on the other hand, discusses just about everything openly. Very few, if any, topics are off limits, and it is quite normal to have family discussions around feelings and emotions. Natalie and I met in college. In workshops, I often (sort of) joke that Natalie taught me it's OK to have feelings. The reality is that she taught me to express how I am feeling and to check in with her and other people I care about to be healthier mentally.

Professionally, my journey into learning about and focusing on social-emotional learning began early in my career as a student teacher. My first assignment was at a middle school, and my mentor teacher was also the school counselor. One morning as we were discussing the lesson ahead, she mentioned that I should be especially gentle with two particular students, a brother and a sister, as the night before, they were kicked out of the house by their parent who had come home drunk. While I was not so naïve to think that this type of thing never happened, it was upsetting that it had happened to students who I worked with on a daily basis.

As my career progressed, teaching at the high school and then the elementary level, I had many, many more experiences that brought to light not only the sometimes challenging situations students live in but also some students' lack of social-emotional skills. Some had difficulty self-managing or developing relationships with peers. Others had developed a variety of skills throughout their lives, including resilience, flexibility, kindness, and empathy.

My wife has worked in the field of mental health throughout her career, including working with foster youth and as a counselor in schools and a therapist in private practice. When our son was six, we decided that we were ready to foster children ourselves. Over the course of several years, my wife and I fostered more than 70 children, usually for short-term respite care. We had several children and young people who returned to stay with us multiple times and a few who stayed for several weeks or months at a time. Because the agency we worked with focused on therapeutic foster care, we fostered youth who had experienced extreme trauma or abuse, had been incarcerated and were transitioning back into the community, or otherwise had behavioral or mental health issues that were fairly extreme.

The children we worked with in foster care were often also in local schools. This experience, and my wife's professional knowledge and expertise in working with youth in crisis, deepened my knowledge about the skills students both have and need to develop to be successful in school and in their lives. Our experience as foster parents and my continued experience in schools helped me better understand how having an asset-based perspective benefits me as well as the children and youth I work with. I learned not to focus on the trauma, abuse, or negative experiences these youth endured. Rather, while acknowledging and taking into account those experiences, I learned to focus on the strengths of the people I work with and help them build the knowledge and skills they need to address their mental health and well-being. Natalie enlightened me to the perspective that healing-focused schools, as opposed to "trauma-informed" schools, switch the paradigm and perspective from one of deficit thinking (trauma informed) to asset thinking (healing focused). Similarly, focusing on people's strengths validates their knowledge and experiences while also acknowledging that it is a normal part of being a human to need support sometimes.

Over time, I began to integrate social-emotional skills into my instruction, including focusing on connecting with each student with whom I worked. I began to incorporate ways to learn more about my students, to have them learn more about me, and to integrate strategies for teaching students self-awareness and self-management. I looked for opportunities for students to collaborate more deeply and to build relationships with others, including those whom they were not necessarily friends with outside of school.

Through my experience working in schools and with teachers, it became increasingly clear that both students and teachers could benefit from learning more about social-emotional learning (SEL) and integrating it more deeply into instruction. I began to dig into the research on SEL and started thinking about additional strategies that educators could integrate easily and consistently into instruction. When the COVID-19 pandemic hit in 2020, the need to integrate social-emotional learning grew exponentially, which is what led me to write this book. As I continue to focus on my own social-emotional development and consider how I integrate and demonstrate social-emotional skills on a daily basis, my goal is to share useful, easy-to-use strategies that will benefit us all and give every person the opportunity to learn skills for being a happy and healthy individual.

The goal of this book is to help you and your students become people who are self-aware, are aware of others and their feelings and emotions, are able to self-regulate and manage emotions in good times and bad, can build and maintain positive relationships with others, and make the best possible decisions.

The focus of **Chapter 1** is building **self-awareness**. In this chapter, we will explore the concept of identity and how it relates to social-emotional learning, as well as learn a variety of strategies for integrating self-awareness into instruction.

The focus of **Chapter 2** is **self-management**. In this chapter, we will look at how to provide opportunities for students to manage their emotions and feelings and self-regulate.

Chapter 3 focuses on **social awareness**. We will learn strategies for building perspective-taking, empathy, and collaboration.

In **Chapter 4**, we will explore how to build **relationship skills** with students, strengthen our relationship with each student, and build and foster relationships among students.

The focus of **Chapter 5** is **responsible decision-making**, in which we will review the decision-making process and discover strategies for explicitly teaching these critical skills to students.

Chapter 6 provides suggestions and strategies for **integrating social-emotional learning** into your regular instruction to promote authentic development of students' SEL skills.

Introduction

What is the goal of education today? Often, people say that the purpose of our education system is to create productive members of society—that students grow into adults who contribute positively to our society in a variety of ways, support themselves financially, pursue interests that make them happy, and follow their civic duties. After all, the United States was founded on the principle of life, liberty, and the pursuit of happiness. Yet for students to become productive members of society, they need to have a set of social and emotional skills to help them navigate challenges in a safe and productive way. Inherent in this is that students learn to work with others, to persevere through challenges, to care and have empathy for others, to be respectful yet assertive when needed, and more. Thus, we must include social-emotional learning in instruction.

Why Social-Emotional Learning?

People face many challenges: mental health issues, including fear, stress, anxiety, and depression; negative childhood experiences and trauma, including physical, emotional, and sexual abuse; the death of loved ones; neglect; and domestic violence. Around the country, communities are seeing higher levels of poverty, family discord and dysfunction, drug/opioid addiction, parents working long hours to make ends meet, insufficient food and poor nutrition, poor school attendance, and high mobility rates. These issues often affect students, and that effect carries over into the school day because students cannot simply leave those issues behind them when they walk through the school doors. Students need skills to learn how to deal with these challenges and overcome the negative effect they can bring.

The National Mental Health Association has found that children and adolescents are facing mental health issues in increasing numbers. Issues of mental health affect approximately one in five youths, and of those children, approximately two thirds are not getting the help they need (Perou et al. 2013). This includes students who may be affected by depression: as many as 1 in 33 children and as many as 1 in 8 adolescents. Children who experience depression are more likely to commit suicide. In fact, according to the Centers for Disease Control and Prevention (n.d.) and the National Institute of Mental Health (n.d.), in 2018, suicide was the second leading cause of death for people ages 10 through 34. Children affected by depression are also more likely to experience depression as adults, are more likely to experience anxiety, and may also experience aches and pains, stomachaches, and headaches.

These data support the idea that people need more mental health support and lead us to wonder what we can do to help young people thrive and build social-emotional skills to make good decisions, deal with adversity, and get additional mental health support when needed.

School + SEL = Success

Many teachers feel that the reason to incorporate social-emotional learning (SEL) into instruction is obvious; they may have seen a rise in bullying, student anxiety, and depression or a general lack of social skills in their students over the past several years or decades. They may point to a lack of respectful discourse in our society regarding important issues. The need for social-emotional learning is evident in many aspects of society.

However, some people feel that parents should be the ones teaching SEL at home. While this argument is valid in that a parent is a child's first teacher, parents and families are already under a lot of pressure today. Many parents are working hard just to make ends meet and are unable to focus deeply on these skills when they are with their children. Some parents lack these skills, as they have never had the opportunity to learn or foster

Given the COVID-19 pandemic, social isolation and anxiety about health and safety have had a massive effect on students, especially as they may have been unable to visit with friends and family; have faced a major shift in behavior, including wearing masks in public and maintaining social distancing; and have grappled with uncertainty over school openings. These changes have increased stress, fear, and anxiety in students and teachers alike.

them throughout their lives. Other parents may not have the research base and teaching skills needed to make these skills explicit to their children.

So what does the research have to say about it? The impact of social-emotional learning has been studied fairly extensively over the years. In general, integrating SEL into instruction has been shown to increase academic achievement by an average of 11 percent. These results are consistent across all grade levels, rural and urban schools, and all school types, including schools with ethnically and racially diverse student populations (Durlak et al. 2011; Taylor et al. 2017). Here are some additional, compelling findings:

A 2011 meta-analysis of 213 studies involving 270,000 students showed that the integration of SEL increased social-emotional skills among students, improved social attitudes and behaviors, increased positive classroom behavior, and decreased emotional distress and conduct problems. This led to an 11 percent gain in academic achievement on standardized tests (Durlak et al. 2011).

A 2017 study involving over 97,000 students in kindergarten through middle school showed increases in academic performance, positive attitudes and behavior, and social-emotional skills and decreases in behavior issues, emotional distress, and drug use. The effects were studied from 6 months to 18 years after SEL programs were instituted. The benefits were the same across socioeconomic and racial groups and geographical boundaries (Taylor et al. 2017).

A 2015 study that controlled for demographics such as socioeconomic status and race and ethnicity found that students with strong SEL skills in kindergarten were more likely to graduate from high school and earn a college degree, and were more likely to have stable employment in young adulthood. In addition, they were less likely to live in public housing, receive public assistance, or be involved with police or be in a detention facility (Jones, Greenberg, and Crowley 2015).

Teachers who possess social-emotional skills are more likely to stay in the classroom and in the field of education, as they are better able to develop and maintain relationships with their students, possess better classroom-management skills, serve as behavioral role models for their students, and can better regulate their emotions (Jennings and Greenberg 2009).

Data released in Illinois showed that approximately 75 percent of students entering kindergarten do not have the necessary skills to be successful, including social-emotional skills, literacy skills, and mathematics skills (Burke 2018). The data show that social-emotional skills were the strongest of the three areas surveyed, with approximately 50 percent of students showing readiness in social-emotional skills based on the Kindergarten Individual Development Survey, developed by WestEd (Burke 2018). While these data are specific to Illinois, and 50 percent is promising, if we consider this as potentially representative of students across the country, it also means that approximately half of your classroom will *not* have the SEL skills needed to be successful.

So when you consider what the research shows about the positive impact of social-emotional learning, it is no wonder that School + SEL = Success!

Defining Social-Emotional Learning

Social-emotional learning, or SEL, can be defined as a process in which people learn to identify, understand, monitor and regulate emotions, develop a positive and healthy identity, develop and maintain strong and healthy relationships, and make good decisions that benefit themselves and the greater good. Teaching social-emotional learning, then, entails helping students attain the knowledge, skills, attitudes, and behaviors that people need to make successful choices. When students have developed social-emotional skills, they are better able to manage their emotions, seek help when needed, develop positive relationships, and problem-solve in difficult situations.

The Five Core Competencies

The Collaborative for Academic, Social, and Emotional Learning (CASEL) has been the leading organization for the advancement of SEL education for more than 25 years. It has identified five core competencies related to SEL that are widely recognized and used in the field of social-emotional learning (CASEL 2021):

- Self-awareness
- Self-management
- Social awareness
- Relationship skills
- Responsible decision-making

Self-Awareness

Self-awareness is the ability to recognize your own feelings, interests, and strengths. When people are self-aware, they know who they are and can recognize, define, and describe their personal and social identities and cultural and linguistic assets, and they can identify and define their emotions accurately. They can identify what triggers their emotions and analyze how their emotions affect others.

Self-Management

Self-management is the ability to manage and control emotions. People with self-management can control and regulate their emotions during both very exciting and difficult situations and handle and respond well to daily stresses. Self-management helps us set plans and work toward goals, overcome obstacles, and monitor progress toward personal and academic goals. Self-management also includes regulating emotions, such as impulses and aggression, and managing personal and interpersonal stress, as well as the ability to control attention. Students who display self-management also show resilience, perseverance, and determination, and they seek help when needed.

Social Awareness

Social awareness is the ability to recognize the perspectives, feelings, and emotions of others. People with social awareness observe, notice, and respond to the emotions and perspectives of others, including people with different cultural backgrounds and contexts. They empathize with others. Social awareness includes considering other people's perspectives and strengths and identifying cues to determine how others feel, predict and evaluate others' emotions and reactions, and respect and empathize with others.

Relationship Skills

Strong relationship skills involve the ability to develop and maintain healthy relationships and resist negative social pressures, resolve interpersonal conflict, and seek help when needed. People with strong relationship skills demonstrate the capacity to work with others in diverse settings, make friends, and engage in collaboration. Respecting diverse viewpoints, communicating effectively, demonstrating cultural responsiveness, providing help to others, and demonstrating leadership are also indicators of effective relationship management.

Responsible Decision-Making

Having responsible decision-making skills means exhibiting ethics and respect when making decisions and keeping physical and mental health and safety in mind. Responsible decision-making involves using critical thinking to identify problems and develop appropriate solutions to those problems. Resisting peer pressure, reflecting on how choices affect others and society, making responsible decisions, and reflecting on and evaluating decision-making processes are all indicators of effective and responsible decision-making skills.

Embedded SEL Skills

Embedded within these competencies are other important skills, and students need a variety of them to be successful in their educational, professional, and personal lives. These include skills such as empathy, compassion, kindness, resilience, perseverance, gratitude, and many others. These key social-emotional concepts will be embedded into our discussions of the five core SEL competencies. It would be remiss, however, to not define these topics and explicitly state their importance to social-emotional learning.

Empathy

Empathy encompasses multiple skills and competencies and is a critical skill in the twenty-first century. Empathy, from the prefix *em–*, meaning "in," and the root *pathos*, meaning "feeling," is the ability to understand and relate to another person's thoughts, emotions, or conditions from that person's perspective. Empathy differs from sympathy. From the prefix *syn–*, meaning "together," *sympathy* relates more to feelings of pity or sorrow for someone else's trouble or grief.

While the definition of empathy seems simple, demonstrating it encompasses several skills. These skills are also embedded in the five core competencies of social-emotional learning. For one, to be empathetic, one needs to be self-aware. Self-awareness encompasses the ability to distinguish your own feelings from the feelings of others. Additionally, social awareness is needed to take others' perspectives into account, including identifying cues to determine how others feel. Empathy is also at the heart of relationship management, as showing empathy helps develop strong relationships. Finally, to demonstrate empathy in a healthy way, we must also demonstrate self-management by regulating our own emotional responses.

Kindness

Kindness is consistently ranked as a key skill for children and adults. Kindness can be defined as having the qualities of and demonstrating friendliness, consideration, and concern for others. People who demonstrate kindness generally do not expect anything in return, such as praise or rewards. Words associated with kindness include *warmth, affection, gentleness, encouragement*, and *caring*.

Research shows that parents and teachers overwhelmingly believe that kindness is an important skill, perhaps even more important than good grades, for students' future success. In a Sesame Workshop survey, 78 percent of teachers and 73 percent of parents surveyed stated that it is more important for their children to be kind than it is for them to be academically successful. Yet 86 percent of teachers and 70 percent of parents surveyed worry that the world is an unkind place for children (Sesame Workshop 2016).

Research suggests that teaching and practicing kindness has many benefits, including reducing bullying in schools. Other benefits include increased meaningful relationships and connections among peers and increased feelings of joy and happiness among students (Layous et al. 2012). Research also shows improved mental health, as being kind increases the release of oxytocin and endorphins in the brain, which can reduce stress, lower blood pressure, and build feelings of optimism and self-worth. The increase of oxytocin, endorphins, and serotonin levels is also related to increased memory and learning, as well as healthy mood, sleep, and digestion (Hamilton 2011).

Resilience

Resilience can be defined as the ability and capacity to cope with, adapt to, and recover from hardship, stressors, crises, or trauma. Resilience in children and adolescents starts with healthy relationships with important adults in their lives. As students build positive experiences over time, their resilience grows. Similarly, when students are allowed and able to cope with more manageable stressors and threats, they build skills and experiences in seeing other stressors as manageable, both physically and mentally. The positive relationships they have with others facilitate learning to cope with the stressors they will encounter in their lives.

Gratitude

The term *gratitude* stems from the Latin word *gratus*, meaning "pleasing or thankful." Many of us think of gratitude as thankfulness or appreciation for someone or something in our lives. This gratitude may be for someone showing us kindness or generosity, for a feeling of stability or good health, for the people who love us and care for and about us, or simply for the beauty we see around us every day. Research indicates that gratitude has a direct and positive correlation to life satisfaction and builds a sense of connection to others (Allen 2018). In addition, noticing, feeling, and expressing gratitude increases satisfaction in many areas of our lives, including school, work, family, community, friends, and ourselves. It also decreases depression and feelings of unhappiness.

Competency Connections

Many years ago, Dr. Hollis Scarborough developed the reading rope infographic, demonstrating how learning to read is composed of several "strands" that are interconnected and interdependent (International Dyslexia Association 2018). As I think about that image, it strikes me that social-emotional learning is similar; the five competencies discussed in this book are intertwined, interconnected, and interdependent. However, rather than a rope that is braided together, the competencies are more like a DNA helix. We cannot completely separate the competencies and isolate them; they rely on one another. The competencies are also interwoven into our being. They make up the social fabric of who we are and how we engage with one another. While it is important to look at individual competencies, we should also look at the whole. The five competencies, as well as related skills and attitudes, such as compassion, empathy, kindness, gratitude, and resilience, all work together to foster well-being.

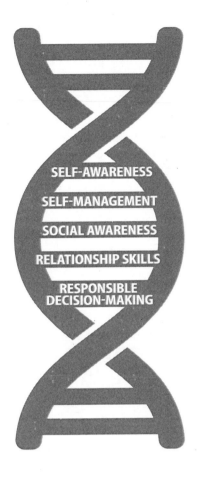

Similarly, we cannot teach the competencies in isolation and should not consider the teaching of SEL as a lesson or two that we deliver throughout the week and then forget about. Rather, SEL is something that should be ingrained in our way of teaching and learning. We want students to learn the content and skills we are teaching. But just as important, we want them to be good people, aware of their feelings and the feelings of others, and aware that their actions affect others and others' actions affect them. We want students to be able to make responsible decisions for their lives and for the betterment of humanity and to have healthy, positive relationships throughout their lives.

Let's look at how these connections play out in our everyday lives. Self-awareness is affected by, and affects, all the competencies directly. For example, self-awareness and self-management are closely tied. As students become more self-aware, they realize how their feelings and emotions manifest in their lives and consider how to respond as needed. Self-management helps students handle the daily stressors of their lives and get through difficult situations. Students self-manage by regulating their emotions, overcoming obstacles, and working toward short- and long-term goals. We also display self-management when we show perseverance and determination and seek help when needed. None of this would be possible without self-awareness.

Self-awareness also leads to social awareness and relationship management. As we become more aware of ourselves, our identities, and our emotional states, it is easier to recognize emotions in others; learn about, respect, and value the identities of others; and have empathy. This, in turn, allows us to build relationships that are healthy and meaningful. For a relationship to work, we must have an awareness of the other person, which includes how they are feeling and how our actions affect them. Through effective communication, we gain deeper awareness and build and foster relationships with other people.

Self-management also leads to more fulfilling and positive relationships. We need to learn to manage our emotions to achieve personal goals and be more successful, personally and socially. If we are unable to manage our own behaviors and ourselves, it will be more difficult for us to manage our relationships.

How can we make responsible decisions if we are unaware of ourselves, our feelings and emotions, and our effect on others? We can't. Without self-awareness, making positive responsible decisions is challenging at best.

Decision-making affects nearly every aspect of our lives. When decisions affect other people, social skills help us as we communicate. Responsible decision-making and social skills, then, go hand-in-hand. As educators, we use social skills on a daily basis to be supportive of students, courteous to parents and colleagues, flexible in our instruction, and responsible for student learning and well-being.

Clearly, the competencies are intertwined, interconnected, and interdependent. It is often hard to consider one without its effects on the others.

Social-Emotional Learning and the Standards

As educators, it is important to consider how SEL fits within the context of what we are expected to teach. As of April 2021, approximately half of the United

States have developed or are developing some form of social-emotional learning standards. (See figure I.1.)

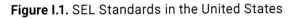

Figure I.1. SEL Standards in the United States

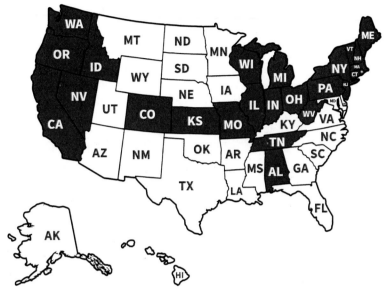

■ States with Social-Emotional Learning Standards in Place or under Development

We can also make connections between SEL and state or national academic standards. While most state and national academic standards do not specifically call out SEL, some standards can be better met when students are improving in the areas of self-management, self-regulation, and responsible decision-making. Additionally, social skills such as perseverance, persistence, and resourcefulness are useful and beneficial as students reach to achieve the rigor of today's academic standards.

I often meet educators who share that they don't feel they have time to integrate SEL because they are trying to help students meet the rigorous academic standards set forth by their states. Yet researchers suggest that learning is 50 percent cognitive and 50 percent social and emotional (Brown, Corrigan, and Higgins-D'Alessandro 2012). Students need to have strong SEL skills to help them tackle new learning, to maintain positive attitudes when learning is challenging, and to interact successfully with classmates and teachers to meet the demands of today's academic standards. For example, mathematics standards and practices require a new level of focus, coherence, and rigor. When students become frustrated or confused by the content, they must persevere to meet the standards. Additionally, English language arts standards require students to interact with more complex text and gather evidence. Students need to be aware of what they do and do not understand about the text and be able to ask for help when they do not understand. For both mathematics and English language arts, students need to have strong communication and collaboration skills as they interact with their teachers and peers.

Consider the standards in figure I.2 and some of the social-emotional skills that could help with their implementation.

Figure I.2. Standards and Social-Emotional Learning Skills

English Language Arts Standards	
Standard	**Necessary SEL Skills**
Analyze how and why individuals, events, or ideas develop and interact over the course of a text.	▸ Label and recognize own and others' emotions ▸ Analyze emotions and how they affect others ▸ Evaluate others' emotional reactions ▸ Reflect on how current choices affect the future
Prepare for and participate effectively in a range of conversations and collaborations with diverse partners, building on others' ideas and expressing their own clearly and persuasively.	▸ Exhibit cooperative learning and work toward group goals ▸ Communicate effectively ▸ Cultivate relationships with those who can be resources when help is needed ▸ Provide help to those who need it ▸ Demonstrate leadership skills when necessary, being assertive and persuasive ▸ Prevent interpersonal conflict but manage and resolve it when it does occur
Mathematics Standards	
Standard	**Necessary SEL Skills**
Make sense of problems and persevere in solving them.	▸ Demonstrate self-efficacy ▸ Work toward goals ▸ Control attention ▸ Regulate emotions ▸ Seek help when needed ▸ Demonstrate perseverance

Construct viable arguments, and critique the reasoning of others.	► Respect others
	► Understand other points of view and perspectives
	► Identify social cues (verbal, physical) to determine how others feel
	► Predict others' feelings and reactions
	► Manage and express emotions in relationships, respecting diverse viewpoints

SEL, Social Justice, and Equity

The complicated nature of race is evident in our society today, as ongoing discussions about racism and racial, social, and educational justice and equity have been integrated into discussions in schools. It is important, then, that we consider the sociopolitical and sociolinguistic realities of our society and the world and how they impact social-emotional learning.

Ignoring the fact that discrimination and prejudice exist is detrimental to students, and no amount of teaching self-awareness or self-management will eliminate that reality. Social-emotional learning should be rooted in the context of the students we serve and in teaching students how we can honor, respect, and celebrate our differences; learn new perspectives; and respond to one another in ways that build us up.

Because of the injustices that exist, we must teach students skills to confront hate, bias, and inequity. Students can start this process by engaging in conversations about these topics. To do this, they will need to be self-aware in terms of their own identities and the various facets that make them who they are, including their racial, ethnic, linguistic, and religious backgrounds. Socially aware people understand that others may have differing backgrounds and cultural perspectives, as well as different ways to approach topics and situations. Teachers and students alike should recognize that culture and identity are at the forefront of how we maintain well-being, the actions we take to cope with difficulties, how we build and maintain positive relationships, and how we recognize and express our emotions.

Dena Simmons (2019) argues that due to the increase in race-based, cultural, and religious-based violence, we must engage students in learning that will allow them to create meaningful change in the world. By building in opportunities for students to engage in conversations about what is happening in their schools, their communities, the country, and the world, they can move toward confronting the injustices in the world and make the world a better place. By teaching the five key competencies of social-emotional learning (self-awareness, self-management, social awareness, relationship skills, and responsible decision-making), we can begin to do just that.

Throughout this book, you will find suggestions and strategies that will help build students' SEL skills while being culturally and linguistically responsive.

Instruction and Social-Emotional Learning

How do we get from where we are to being more inclusive, asset-based educators who truly hold unconditional positive regard for students? One way to begin is through embedding social-emotional learning into our instruction every day. Through the integration of specific strategies from this book—many of which are short and require little preparation—we begin to move toward embedding social-emotional competencies into everything we do in our classrooms. We develop deeper emotional intelligence and generally become happier and better regulated as we see these skills manifest in our own lives. Teaching something is often the best way to learn it deeply. As we teach students about SEL through embedding specific strategies in the classroom, we see growth not only in their skills but also in ourselves. From there, SEL becomes a way of being, a way we walk through the world, how we interact and build relationships with others, how we express ourselves, and how we cope with difficult times.

Strategies Lead to a Way of Being

In schools, the integration of SEL includes teaching students what the five core competencies are as well as the skills and behaviors associated with them. Through the integration of SEL instruction, teachers help students practice SEL competencies in a safe environment in the classroom, pointing out when the skills are being used effectively and when they need to be incorporated more deeply. Instruction in the actions and language associated with these topics benefits students as they navigate the world.

However, instruction is not enough. The core competencies are not discrete lessons and skills that students should learn about and practice only during a morning meeting, homeroom, or advisory period. SEL should be more than lessons that are then forgotten during the rest of the day. SEL competencies and skills, as well as other key practices such as empathy, gratitude, and kindness, are a way of being. They inform how we move through the world, how we interact with others, and how we carry ourselves.

Positive Classroom Environment

Children are not born knowing how to navigate the wide range of emotions they feel on a day-to-day basis. In a blog post titled "Seven Surprising Facts About Emotions that Every Child Needs to Know," Ann Douglas (2016) shares facts about emotions in ways that are easy for students to understand. Helping students navigate these emotions and understand them can lead to a positive classroom environment.

1. **Different people show their emotions in different ways.** Different people may respond differently to the same or similar situations, and this is one of the things that makes life so interesting!

2. **Looks can be deceiving.** Just because someone looks angry or happy, they may not actually feel that particular emotion. People mask or hide emotions at times for certain reasons, such as when you respond to a loved one giving you a hideous garment as a gift. Children should consider, though, the effect this action may have.

3. **There are many spheres of influence.** Emotions can be triggered by something from within or outside your control. Sometimes emotions are triggered by a past experience or by the context in which the emotion is happening.

4. **Mild, medium, or hot?** Emotions can be experienced in varying levels of intensity, just like hot sauce. There are many different levels of emotions, both positive and negative, and people have developed language that indicates the level of intensity of particular emotions.

5. **Take it up a notch, or take it down a notch.** An emotion can become more intense or less intense, depending on what else is going on. Emotions can build on each other and cause feelings to intensify, or a situation or words from another person may help cancel out the initial emotion. This can work in both positive and negative ways.

6. **Emotions come in complex combinations.** It is possible, and even likely, to feel varying emotions simultaneously, including sometimes feeling emotions

that seem like opposites. Excitement can coincide with anxiety, for example. People may experience this when starting at a new school or when interviewing for a job.

7. **Regulating emotions is an ongoing process.** The skill of self-regulation does not necessarily come easily. As our emotional lives become more complex, we need to continue to practice and acquire the skills to make our emotions work for us, not against us. (Adapted from Douglas 2016)

Social-emotional learning works best when the classroom is a place of positive learning experiences and relationships. When teachers focus on positives, they are friendly, enjoy themselves and their students, and are dedicated to pointing out what students are doing well as opposed to what students are doing wrong. This takes effort and does not mean that we let students behave inappropriately or do whatever they want. It begins with having an unconditional positive regard for students.

Beginning with this stance will benefit us when we encounter behaviors and personalities that we are uncomfortable with. When we see students behaving in a way that we feel is counterproductive, we can address the behavior, focusing on the behavior rather than on the student. This teaches students that they will be respected even when their behaviors or actions are not appropriate. This allows students to understand that you care about them, respect them, and want them to learn and grow. It shows that you know everyone makes mistakes.

Educating the whole child depends on ensuring that students learn in caring, supportive, safe, and empowering settings. For true learning to take place, students must feel safe to take risks, safe to share ideas, and safe to make mistakes—a well-managed classroom supports these things. Creating this environment requires that teachers build a positive classroom culture that embraces risk in learning, collaboration, and celebration of the learning process. If students feel they will be embarrassed when asking questions, attempting to solve problems, or being creative, the learning process will be hampered.

A positive classroom community is asset-based rather than deficit-based. In addition to holding students in a positive light, we should focus on students' strengths while looking at areas of improvement. Occasionally, there is a focus on what is wrong, such as poor behaviors, trauma, or low academic performance. When we use asset-based thinking, we consider the strengths students bring—their resilience, their sense of humor, the relationships they have, their creativity—and build on those strengths as students continue to develop social-emotional skills.

Consider the shift from deficit-based to asset-based language and thinking:

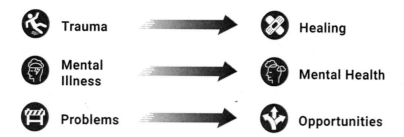

This simple shift in language sends a powerful message to students, youth, and the community: You are more than your experiences. While those experiences are important to know and understand, the focus is on healing and well-being, not on the issues themselves.

Stop and Reflect

1. Think about a student you currently work with. How might that student benefit from the integration of SEL into your instruction?

2. Describe the culture in your classroom. Are students willing and able to take risks in learning? When a student makes a mistake, how do other students react? How do you handle students who tease other students who make mistakes?

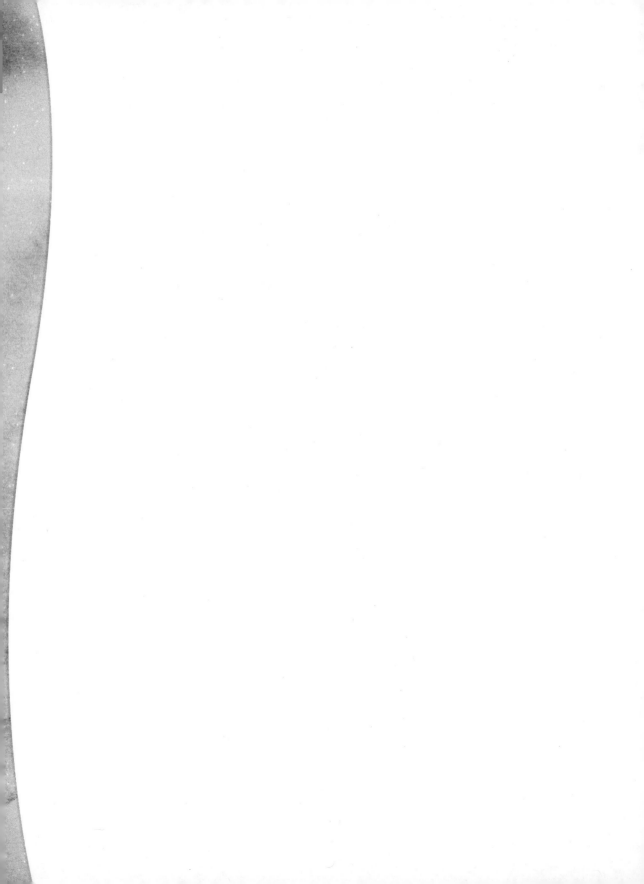

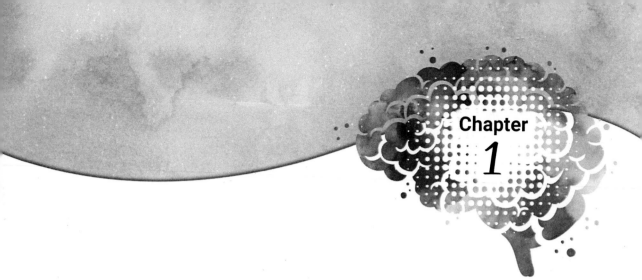

Self-Awareness

Think back to a time when you went to the doctor for a checkup. The doctor likely began with a question such as "How are you?" or "How are things going?" Your response played a critical role in the doctor's reply. As you shared specific areas of concern, the doctor could consider if any treatments were needed or if any follow-up questions were required to pinpoint the exact issue. However, if you were unaware of any specific health issues you were experiencing, it would have been difficult for the doctor to provide the care or treatment you needed. Your self-awareness allowed you to describe what you were feeling and helped the doctor resolve your health concerns.

Similarly, as school professionals, we sometimes need to determine what is happening with a student and understand their feelings and emotional state. A student's emotional state affects their learning and their willingness and ability to engage in educational activities. When students are unaware of their emotional states and are unable to communicate how they feel, it is more difficult to provide engaging and exciting instruction or to be responsive to students' needs.

Defining Self-Awareness

Self-awareness is the ability to recognize one's own feelings and emotions, interests, strengths, values, beliefs, and personal and social identities. People are self-aware when they can identify and recognize specific emotions, express what triggers those emotions, and analyze and understand how their emotions affect others. When people are self-aware, they recognize their strengths in terms of their personalities, characters, and personal and social identities and use those strengths to navigate the world.

Being self-aware has many benefits. As we learn to recognize who we are and how we feel at any given time—in both our physical and emotional states—we are better able to navigate the complexities of life. For example, when we are able to recognize that we feel frustrated, we can take actions to de-escalate those feelings so that we don't make a situation worse. Additionally, if we recognize what actions make us happy and content, we can look for opportunities to engage in those actions more often. Self-awareness is the precursor to what many students must be explicitly taught: self-management. We will delve more deeply into self-management in the next chapter, but we begin here to see the interwoven nature of SEL.

Self-awareness may be easy for students from environments where discussing feelings is common. Some people discuss their feelings on a regular basis, checking in with others about how they feel in any given moment. Through simple check-ins such as "How are you feeling?" people share their emotional state, which helps the person being asked to be more self-aware and creates awareness for the person asking the question. Other people rarely consider their own feelings in a deep or meaningful way, living their lives by reacting to the feelings that arise but not thinking about how they feel or why. This can create a level of chaos in people's lives, as they do not realize what their emotional states are in any given moment.

Identity: A Key Aspect of Self-Awareness

Being self-aware includes knowing the various aspects of our identity. Identity can be defined as who we are as individuals; it includes such things as ethnicity, gender, race, national origin, sexual orientation, age group, ability or disability, religion, and socioeconomic status. These aspects of identity influence our values and norms to some degree and may affect our behavior. The topic of identity, then, is critical as we consider the five competencies. We will begin by considering both our own identities and how we can validate students' identities and support them in being themselves completely and authentically.

It may be more appropriate to discuss our *identities* as opposed to our *identity*, as no one is singular in identity. Sometimes, our different identities may appear to be in conflict. A person might be devoutly religious while also LGBTQIA+. Or a person might identify as Jewish but celebrate both Hanukkah and Christmas with family and friends. Other identities, such as national origin, may be complicated, as in a case where someone was born in one country but lives in another country.

Consider each of the following aspects of identity from your own perspective and from students' perspectives. Note that not all aspects of identity are listed; however, these are some of the more commonly discussed identities.

Ethnicity

Ethnicity refers to cultural background or traditions that are shared among a group. Aspects of ethnicity include language, food, dress, stories, art, and music. Ethnicity also affects behaviors and ideas such as how to demonstrate respect, gender expectations, concept of time, and ideals such as fairness and justice. It is important to note that ethnicity and race are not the same and that race should not be used to refer to ethnicity.

Gender

Historically, gender identity has referred to traditional roles and behaviors of females and males in a society. However, many gender identities are recognized today, including but not limited to male, female, transgender, nonbinary, pangender, agender, and cisgender. People may identify with any of these gender identities, regardless of the gender they were assigned at birth.

Race

Race often is an important part of our identity. Yet race is an arbitrary label that has no scientific basis. The idea of race has been imposed based on observable physical traits and can be defined as a socially constructed story of human geography and denotable phenotypes.

Nationality

Our national identity is usually based on where we were born or where we live. As mentioned previously, people can also identify with more than one country, especially if they were born in one country and live in another, or if they were born in one country but their family or ancestors are from another country.

Sexual Orientation

Sexual orientation is an important aspect of our identities. People may identify as heterosexual, gay, lesbian, bisexual, pansexual, or asexual.

Age

Age also influences our identity. One may identify as a child, a teenager, a 20-something, middle-aged, an older adult, and so on. The way people dress and communicate, what they talk about, and the activities they enjoy often relate to their age or life stage.

Ability/Disability

A person's abilities and disabilities affect identity. The idea of "disability identity" refers to people with a disability having a positive outlook toward themselves and a positive connection to the disability community. A disability identity can help people develop a positive self-concept, help affirm their disabilities, and build self-worth and pride.

Religion

Religion or spirituality often plays a very strong role in a person's identity. People's religious beliefs may influence a variety of aspects of their lives, including their daily choices and how they communicate with and treat others.

Socioeconomic Status

Our identities can also be tied to our socioeconomic status, which has to do with our societal class and may be tied to our careers or earning power. Socioeconomic status can also influence our values and behavior (Manstead 2018). For example, it may affect attitudes about how success is achieved.

Building a Sense of Self

When we are self-aware and value our own identities, we are more likely to be open to and validate the identities of others. We must first begin by considering our own identities and deepening our own self-awareness as adults who work with children and young adults. When we do this, we also develop empathy for others, as we are better able to walk in their shoes. This may be the first time you have deeply considered all the aspects of your identity, or you may be very self-aware in terms of your identity.

As teachers, building self-awareness around students' identities is crucial. When we do, we demonstrate to students that they are important and valued for who they are. We also help develop empathy in students—a critical skill in our diverse world. Young people are often still formulating and developing their identities, and we can support them in developing a positive sense of self through self-awareness.

Teaching self-awareness relies heavily on reflection, language, dialogue, and vocabulary instruction. For students to develop deep self-awareness of their identities, emotions, and feelings, they need to learn to productively express themselves—either visually or through words and phrases that provide precision and nuance—describing who they are and how they feel. Therefore, language is a critical aspect of the work that has to be done. Just as young students name their emotions using words such as *happy*, *sad*, or *mad*, they describe their identities in relatively simplistic ways as well, using words such as *boy*, *girl*, *kid*, and so on. In upper elementary school, students begin to use more sophisticated language to describe their feelings, using words such as *frustrated*, *upset*, and *excited*. They begin to explore their identities and describe them more accurately. As students reach the secondary level, they consider how emotions and feelings affect their actions and learn vocabulary to help them identify and more deeply understand what is happening, which will ultimately lead them to deeper levels of self-management and self-regulation.

Who Am I?

The Who Am I activity has students share information about themselves, including descriptions of their families, foods and activities they like/dislike, music or books they enjoy, and significant events in their lives. This get-to-know-you activity is an important aspect of building a community of learners that is founded on respect, diversity, and self-awareness.

These sample questions provide a surface-level understanding of students—who they are and the roles they play as individuals within their various communities. To deepen self-awareness, we can have students consider additional aspects of themselves, such as their personalities and character traits and the various aspects of their identities discussed previously.

Sample Questions, Statements, and Topics for a *Who Am I?* Project

- My name is _____.
- My name means _____.
- I want to be called _____.
- I use the pronouns _____.
- My family members include _____.
- Some of my friends are _____.
- I live in _____.
- I have also lived in _____.
- My birthday is _____.

- My favorite food is _____.
- My favorite color is _____.
- My favorite movie/TV show is _____.
- My favorite book is _____.
- My favorite song is _____.
- My favorite sport/game is _____.
- My favorite quote is _____.
- My favorite animal is _____.
- For fun, I like to _____.

Have students use graphic organizers or create posters to share the information about themselves. Other creative formats that link to content areas such as music, art, and graphic design are shown below. For an added challenge, have students choose from the list, or have them suggest their own creative ideas for expressing who they are. Most of the ideas can be adapted for any grade level.

Sample *Who Am I?* Project Ideas

Grades K–2	Grades 3–5	Grades 6–12
time capsule	riddle	time line
comic strip	video	biography
scrapbook	song	sitcom script
collage	presentation	newspaper article
rhyming book	brochure	short story
illustrated book	commercial	play script
sculpture	letter	flowchart

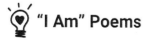 **"I Am" Poems**

Creating "I Am" poems allows students to focus both on social-emotional skills and language arts skills. For example, students can be taught about figurative language and embed it into their poems. Personification, alliteration, imagery, mood, simile, and metaphor are all examples of language tools that students can incorporate into their "I Am" poems. For an added interesting element, consider having bilingual students write their poems in their home languages. Many poetry styles lend themselves well to "I Am" poems, including acrostic, alphabet poem, quatrain or cinquain, diamante, concrete, haiku, limerick, or a poem for two voices.

 ## My Heart Map

In this activity, students fill in a heart shape with words, colors, and/or pictures that celebrate their identities. Using the aspects of identity shared previously, students can divide the heart into larger and smaller sections and fill in those sections based on how strongly they feel a connection to each aspect of their identities.

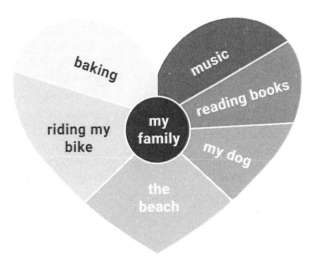

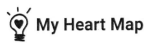 ## The Identity Pyramid

In this activity, students describe aspects of their identities and show how those aspects manifest more dominantly or more subtly. Begin by teaching students about the various aspects of identity described previously. Which specific aspects you choose may depend on the grade level you teach. Students rank the aspects of their identities and stack them in a pyramid based on their importance in their lives. More than one aspect of a person's identity can be placed on each level of the pyramid.

Other shapes and design elements can be used as well. For example, students can make bubbles, circles, or diamonds and use colors and words to show the various aspects of their identities.

Identifying Personality Traits and Character Strengths

Researchers have found that five major personality traits influence the way people feel, behave, and think. These five traits are openness, conscientiousness, extroversion, agreeableness, and neuroticism. Figure 1.1 shows each of these traits, as well as their indicators. The indicators are represented on a scale that demonstrates the range of feelings, behaviors, and thoughts associated with the personality trait.

Figure 1.1. The Five Major Personality Traits and Their Indicators

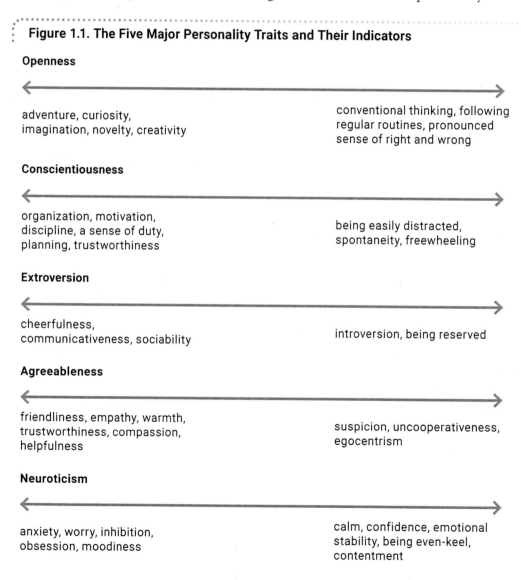

Openness

adventure, curiosity, imagination, novelty, creativity

conventional thinking, following regular routines, pronounced sense of right and wrong

Conscientiousness

organization, motivation, discipline, a sense of duty, planning, trustworthiness

being easily distracted, spontaneity, freewheeling

Extroversion

cheerfulness, communicativeness, sociability

introversion, being reserved

Agreeableness

friendliness, empathy, warmth, trustworthiness, compassion, helpfulness

suspicion, uncooperativeness, egocentrism

Neuroticism

anxiety, worry, inhibition, obsession, moodiness

calm, confidence, emotional stability, being even-keel, contentment

Character traits fit within these personality traits and provide us with insights into people's behaviors. Figure 1.2 shows a variety of character traits that represent students' potential strengths. Depending on students' grade level, less desirable or more negative traits can be included. For example, students might consider how they can improve on traits such as being absent-minded, stingy, suspicious, or quick-tempered.

Figure 1.2. Positive Character Traits

accessible	dynamic	organized
adaptable	efficient	passionate
affable	energetic	perceptive
affectionate	enthusiastic	persuasive
amusing	focused	polite
articulate	gracious	quiet
clever	honest	rational
confident	humorous	reliable
courageous	idealistic	resourceful
creative	independent	responsible
daring	innovative	sensible
decisive	intuitive	sensitive
dependable	inventive	sincere
determined	meticulous	spontaneous
diligent	optimistic	tolerant

All people have specific strengths that they bring with them to every situation. When people know their character strengths, they can apply them to help them improve relationships, solve problems, and enhance their well-being. This is true for students and teachers alike. With students, we can help them deepen their own self-awareness by having them consider their personality traits and character strengths. When we understand students' strengths, we can use this information to improve engagement in learning; help them navigate the complexities of their lives in the classroom, on the playground, and in their communities; and more deeply understand their own actions and motivations. As teachers, when we know our character strengths, we can analyze those strengths and use them to improve instruction, as well as our relationships with students.

Teaching about character traits involves defining the words and helping students understand the sometimes subtle differences between them. Student-friendly definitions, pictures and sketches, or synonyms and antonyms are useful tools. Analyzing characters in books and novels or people from history, for example, can point out how a person's repeated actions reveal a particular character trait.

 ## Character Trait Bingo

Begin with sets of character trait cards. Each card should list a character trait, a student-friendly definition, and an image that represents the character trait. Each student playing needs a set of cards. Students sort the trait cards into four categories: a lot like me, somewhat like me, not much like me, and not at all like me. Alternatively, students can color a list of character traits using the stoplight highlight or coloring technique, where they color each trait with a color: green—a lot like me, yellow—somewhat like me, orange—not much like me, and red—not at all like me (or any color variation of your choosing).

Once students have the traits sorted, they take the "a lot like me" and "somewhat like me" categories and fill in a blank bingo grid with the specific character traits. Students should randomly place the traits in the bingo grid. If they don't have enough traits from the two categories listed, they can add traits from the other categories.

Then play bingo. The caller—either the teacher or another student—says the name of the trait and the definition, or for an added challenge, reads only the definition. When students mark horizontal, vertical, or diagonal lines, they call out "Bingo!" and win the game. Blackout bingo, in which all the spaces must be marked to win, is a fun alternative.

 ## Demonstrating Character

During this activity, students consider how character traits are demonstrated by people's actions and words.

To begin, have students choose a character trait that they feel comes easily to them. Over the course of a day or a week (or a month for older students), have students record the actions they take and the words they say that they feel show that character trait.

Students then choose a character trait that they would like to exemplify or demonstrate more often. Have students brainstorm actions that would show that specific character trait. Each day or week, students choose from the list of actions and work to demonstrate the trait.

As an alternative, students can record their actions over the course of a day or week (or a month for older students) and analyze them to infer the character traits they demonstrated.

See the Digital Resources for graphic organizers students can use to determine the relationship between character traits and actions.

Demonstrating Character Graphic Organizers

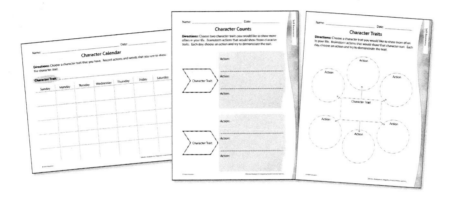

Identifying and Naming Feelings

A key step in building self-awareness is being able to identify and name how we feel. Naming feelings and understanding the gradations that the names of feelings represent will help students understand their own feelings. Consider the following adjectives and the feelings they represent:

- ▶ happy, content, gleeful, ecstatic, joyful, amused
- ▶ angry, enraged, upset, frustrated, aggressive, irritated, resentful
- ▶ sad, lonely, vulnerable, depressed, isolated, remorseful
- ▶ scared, anxious, insecure, humiliated, frightened, terrified
- ▶ surprised, excited, startled, perplexed, astonished

Students can and should learn the names of various emotions, especially the nuanced meanings and gradations of feelings. For example, happiness can relate to a variety of feelings, but if students don't have those adjectives in their vocabularies, they cannot describe the specific types of happiness they are feeling. These words provide specificity to the feelings or emotions experienced.

It is important to avoid labeling feelings as good or bad and instead refer to them as comfortable or uncomfortable. By using this language, we begin to understand that emotions of sadness or anger may not feel comfortable, but they are a normal part of the human experience. They are like signposts guiding us to turn left, turn right, stop, or go. In essence, these feelings show us that we may need to change course.

Figure 1.3 lists feelings words that are separated by grade-level bands. The lists are not exhaustive and are simply guides to words that may be most appropriate to teach at different grade bands. This is not to say that students cannot learn words from lists for other grade bands. Any feelings words can be taught to any group of students, if appropriate and desired. Consider how the word will benefit students and help them more deeply develop self-awareness through understanding feelings.

Tip!

There are many resources available to teach students about feelings and emotions. Here are a few:

- "How Are You Feeling Today?" posters have pictures with labels naming the represented feelings.

- The Feelings Inventory by the Center for Nonviolent Communication lists words that can be used to express a combination of feelings and physical responses.

- Emotion Wheels describe basic emotions and can be used to identify emotions and help people accept how they are feeling.

Figure 1.3. Sample Feeling Words

Grades K–2

brave	disrespected	shy	powerful
cheerful	frustrated	angry	playful
bored	embarrassed	calm	hopeful
confused	silly	happy	loving
surprised	excited	sad	respectful
curious	uncomfortable	scared	important
proud	fantastic	hurt	frightened
disappointed	friendly	mad	worried

Grades 3–5

stubborn	tense	frustrated	terrified
generous	lonely	powerless	furious
ignored	joyful	empty	hesitant
satisfied	excited	inspired	worthless
impatient	amazed	open	insignificant
safe	proud	courageous	inadequate
important	guilty	confident	guilty
relieved	accepted	amused	abandoned
peaceful	startled	energetic	loving
jealous	anxious	eager	confused
overwhelmed	rejected	shocked	awful

Grades 6–8

optimistic	vulnerable	disillusioned	suspicious
insecure	inferior	dismayed	skeptical
submissive	abandoned	inadequate	sarcastic
humiliated	isolated	alienated	judgmental
threatened	apathetic	withdrawn	hateful

Continued

aggressive	sensitive	devastated	repugnant
distant	provocative	insecure	revulsed
critical	fulfilled	jealous	detested
disapproving	inquisitive	resentful	averse
avoiding	ecstatic	enraged	irritated
despairing	liberated	provoked	perplexed
remorseful	in awe	hostile	victimized
ashamed	astonished	infuriated	
indifferent	ridiculed	loathing	

 Feelings Vocabulary Match

Because naming emotions is largely a vocabulary learning exercise, effective vocabulary learning techniques can be applied to help students learn the words. For example, find pictures or representations of specific emotions and print them on cardstock. On another sheet of cardstock, print the names of the feelings or emotions. Cut out the pictures and the word cards (or have students cut them out), and then have students work in pairs or small groups to match the pictures or representations with the names of the emotions. Students should divide the pictures and words evenly and take turns matching and then justifying their matches. Then students can and should use the pictures and words as they discuss the feelings, emotions, and reactions in characters of the stories, novels, or videos they are using. Naming the emotions of others, especially those who appear in text or on video, provides practice for students in a way that is safe and absent of negative consequences. This practice will help students learn to name their own emotions.

 Make an Emotion Book

An emotion book is filled with pages that represent emotions and things that spark those feelings. Students use pictures that they draw, cut from magazines, or print out to create a collage. Each page represents a specific feeling or emotion. Once students have added the pictures or drawings, they should write about the things that inspire these feelings in them. Or they can add additional pictures, drawings, or sketches to each page. Over time, this book can be added to and may change based on students' experiences. In addition, students can add more complex emotions as they understand nuance and distinguish between related emotions, such as happy and elated.

Alternatively, have small groups, pairs, or individuals create pages or short books on one specific emotion or one range of related emotions. These pages could then be compiled into one book or a collection of books and added to the class library. Students can use the books to reflect on current feelings or to look for ways to change their current emotional states.

Emotions Weather Report

In an Emotions Weather Report, students use the weather to describe their feelings. Have students brainstorm a list of different weather. For added comprehension, show students pictures or videos of different types of weather. Once the list is developed, have students consider how the weather represents their feelings. Help students equate different feelings and emotions to each type of weather and add these to the list.

Examples:

- ▶ winds = change
- ▶ rain = tears
- ▶ fog = tired, fuzzy brain, confused
- ▶ tornado = overwhelmed
- ▶ blizzard = outgoing
- ▶ drizzle = timid

When students have a list of weather and corresponding emotions, they can begin their weather reports. These can be done as a quick-write, wherein students represent how they are feeling through a news-style report, or they can draw pictures that represent their feelings through the weather. Students can also do daily check-ins, where they place their name cards, or cards with their initials, on a chart that shows different types of weather. This serves as a tool for self-awareness and is an indicator to the teacher of how each student is feeling. This can be done anonymously; however, you will need to pay attention as students put their magnets or sticky notes in specific categories so that you are aware of their feelings.

Naming Triggers

Once students can name and understand the variety of emotions that they might feel, they can use self-reflection to begin to understand what causes their undesirable feelings. Emotional triggers are the challenges, situations, and people that cause us to feel frustrated, angry, or upset. Almost anything could be an emotional trigger for students. For example, students may feel a great deal of anxiety around tasks they must complete in class. Others may feel triggered by people with whom they have had negative experiences. Specific places where students have experienced trauma can be triggers and bring up feelings of fear or anxiety, even if the trauma happened long ago.

When these triggers occur, not only can uncomfortable feelings arise, such as fear, anger, frustration, or embarrassment, but students' reactions to those triggers can lead to actions such as freezing up, arguing, or saying something they will later regret. Being aware of triggers allows students to acknowledge that everybody has them and that they are part of being human. It also allows students to reflect on how these triggers affect them and, perhaps more important, how their reactions may lead to outcomes that are undesirable. Naming a trigger can look like this: "This is a trigger for me. I thought about this the other day. I'm going to react differently this time." Once students have named it, they can decide how to react. We can help students use self-reflection to think through the choices they have in responding to the trigger. Over time, when encountering and naming triggers, students will have better control of their reactions.

Using Self-Reflection as a Tool

Self-reflection is a tool for teachers and students alike. As teachers, we can use self-reflection in a variety of ways, including considering the level of success of our lessons and how our own actions affect students' emotional well-being. Self-reflection can be challenging for teachers because of the lack of time. However, carving out at least five minutes a day to practice self-reflection can be a good start. The following questions may be helpful:

- ▸ What went well today?
- ▸ When were students at their best today?
- ▸ What contributed to students being at their best?
- ▸ What specific words or actions did I take when students were at their best?

- How did my words or actions contribute to students being at their best?
- When was student classwork or behavior less desirable?
- What contributed to students' exhibiting less than desirable behavior?
- What specific words or actions did I take?
- How did my words or actions contribute to the situation?
- How did I feel when...?
- What did I do or say when I was feeling...?

Just as we engage in self-reflection, we can ask students to engage in self-reflection, too. The questions above can be adapted for students. Students can use the questions for discussions in pairs or small groups, in quick-writes, exit slips, and so on.

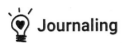

Journaling

Journaling is a tried-and-true writing activity. Teachers at many grade levels use journaling, with or without specific prompts. The prompts previously listed under Using Self-Reflection as a Tool can be modified for students to focus on self-reflection and self-awareness. To vary journaling, use a variety of writing techniques. For example, have students write letters to their past or future selves, sharing how they are feeling today and how they arrived at that feeling.

Sample Grades K–2 Prompts

- What are three things you like to do?
- Tell about a time you felt happy today.
- Tell about a time you felt sad or mad today.
- What is your favorite _____ (*color, animal, game*, etc.), and why?

Sample Grades 3–5 Prompts

- What are two things that make you really happy?
- What do you do when you are feeling good?
- Who is your favorite person, and why?
- What is something you could say to or do for a friend when they are feeling bad?

Sample Grades 6–8 Prompts

▸ If I could say one thing to _____ (my mom, my dad, my best friend, etc.), I would tell them _____.

▸ How do you know how you are feeling? What ways do you display your emotions?

▸ How does _____ (happiness, sadness, anger, excitement, etc.) feel in your body?

▸ What is something you used to love to do but you don't do anymore?

Sample High School Prompts

▸ What is one thing you would do if you knew you could not fail?

▸ What are two things that really annoy you? How do you react when you encounter them?

▸ What is something you need to let go of?

▸ What is something negative you say to yourself that you don't tell anyone? Write a dialogue responding to that voice.

Dialogue journals are a form of interactive journaling. In a dialogue journal, you have a written conversation with the student. After students have written their journal entries, collect the journals and provide responses. It can be helpful to ask a question or two so that students can respond. Questions about self-awareness and how students are feeling can be included in the written conversations.

 Visualize It!

Visualization is a powerful tool that supports self-awareness in several ways. Students can visualize what a desired outcome looks like and work toward making that a reality by making changes to their behaviors. Visualizing the end goal and the steps needed to get there can help make the management of those steps more realistic and less daunting for students.

To help students understand this strategy, start by defining *visualization* as "picturing in your mind's eye what something looks like." Here are simple steps to help students visualize:

1. **Picture familiar items in their minds.** Start with very simple concepts for young students, such as an apple or an orange, a tree, a dog, or a cat. You can invite students to close their eyes to visualize, but this should not be required.

2. **Use a passage of text.** Literature and informational texts are rich sources for visualization. Introductory paragraphs in informational text or passages in literature that describe the setting or a character can be fantastic tools to encourage visualization.

3. **Sketch or draw what they visualize.** This allows students to make the abstract more concrete. Remind them that their drawings or sketches need not be perfect but rather general representations of what they visualized.

4. **Brainstorm and then visualize goals.** Have students consider goals they want to accomplish, both short-term and long-term, and help them visualize the goals they have set.

5. **Determine the steps needed.** Have students consider and write, sketch, or draw the steps they need to take to help realize the goals they have set.

💡 Time Log

A time log is a tool to help determine how students spend their time and how the time spent affects their abilities to accomplish their tasks. The purpose of the time log is to help students learn to manage their time better. Filling in a time log takes dedication, especially if students are to accurately determine how their time is being spent. For younger students, consider keeping a class log based on the agenda or the important tasks that need to be done each day. The younger the students, the shorter the time frame should be, so that students can accurately reflect on how they spend their time. Older students can make a more detailed log of their days, with as much accuracy as possible to determine how they spend their time.

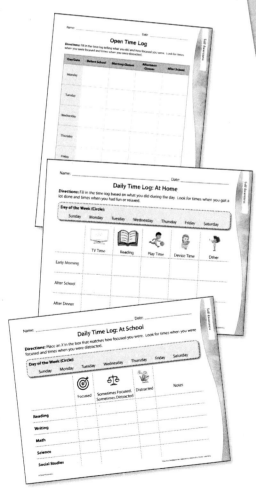

Some students are unaware of how long they spend doing a particular activity. A time log can be completed and analyzed to determine times when students are most productive or when they are easily distracted. This is more manageable if done for short, designated periods of time. For example, students can keep a time log for a week and then take a look at where time spent is out of balance. Have students discuss and make recommendations to one another with the goal of using time more wisely. Sample time logs are provided in the Digital Resources.

Pluses and Deltas

In this activity, students consider what went well and what they would like to change about their own actions or behaviors during lessons. Start by giving each student two 3 x 3 sticky notes, preferably two different colors. On one note, have students draw plus signs. Then have them write about positive aspects of their experiences during the lesson. This could be a time they were especially successful, a time they persevered, or another positive aspect; they should describe their behaviors or feelings during that time. On the second note, have students draw triangles, which represent delta, or change. On this note, have students write things they would like to change from the lesson regarding their feelings or, more specifically, the behaviors they engaged in based on those feelings.

Pass the Ball

Start by having small groups of students stand in circles. Explain that they will be asked a series of questions, and the student with the ball (or other soft object) will answer the question. When the student has finished answering the question, they will pass the ball to the next person, who then answers the same question. As an alternative, have the next student respond by summarizing briefly what the previous student said. For fun, students can toss the ball to someone else in the circle rather than pass it to the person next to them.

Sample Questions

- ▶ What did you like best about this activity/lesson? Why?
- ▶ What did you like least about this activity/lesson? Why?
- ▶ What did you learn by participating in this activity/lesson?
- ▶ What are two or three words you can use to describe how you feel about this activity/lesson?
- ▶ What are some other related activities/lessons that you would like to do?

- ▸ Why was it important that we worked together to complete this activity/lesson?
- ▸ What, if anything, will you do differently because of the experiences you had while participating in this activity/lesson?
- ▸ Would you like to participate in this activity/lesson again? Why or why not?
- ▸ If we did this activity/lesson again, what could we do to make it better?

As an alternative, you can use beach balls for this activity. Rather than posing a question that all students begin with, write questions on each colored section of the beach balls. As students stand in small groups, they toss the balls around. You can have students hit or toss the beach ball three times, with the fourth person catching the ball. That student then answers the question on the section that lands on his or their right (or left) hand. As an alternative, you can write questions all over the ball and have students answer the questions that are closest to the finger you indicate. After answering the question, the student tosses the ball, and students hit the ball three times, with the fourth person catching the ball and answering the next question (adapted from the Center on the Social and Emotional Foundations for Early Learning n.d.).

Letter to a Future Student

The Letter to a Future Student is a reflective writing activity designed to be used at the end of a learning period, such as after the first 100 days of school, at the end of a quarter or semester, at the end of a unit of study, or at the end of the year. In this activity, students reflect on the unit/course and their time in the classroom. The letter can include a number of prompts, such as important learning, how the unit/course will impact them in the future, how the information relates to the world at large, what they wish they had known going into the unit/course that they now know, or what was especially interesting, important, or challenging to them personally. Have students include tips or advice to future students as well.

This simple self-reflection activity serves as a way for students to consider their own growth and can be an assessment of learning and growth for the teacher, while allowing students to practice and improve their writing skills.

Metaphoric Metamorphosis

This end-of-learning activity, to be used after a powerful unit or at the end of a term or course, is a fun way to have students reflect on how they have changed over the course of the learning period. This activity builds self-awareness and creativity in students. Take the following steps to lead students through this activity.

1. Ask students to consider their transformations over the learning period. What do they know now that they did not know before the lesson(s)? Why is the information important to them? How does having this information affect their futures in terms of learning, career goals, and so on?

2. Present the concept of metaphor if students are unfamiliar with it. Explain that they will consider their own changes as metaphors, such as superpowers, gardens, or scientific phenomena.

3. Share your own example of a metaphor that represents a change in your life. This will serve as a model for students as they consider their own changes and develop their own metaphors.

4. Have students create their own metaphors, either through writing or as artistic endeavors. Giving students choice in this area provides them with opportunities to be creative and have fun, while playing to their strengths. Students might create written stories, create videos, make sculptures, create comic strips, or paint scenes.

Reflecting on Uncomfortable Feelings

Emotions, especially uncomfortable emotions, play a powerful role in our lives. Humans have a negativity bias; we are more likely to remember uncomfortable situations as a survival skill. For example, if we eat something that makes us ill, we are more likely to remember it so as to avoid the food in the future. Similarly, when we find ourselves in a precarious situation, such as when we climb a tall ladder, we may feel anxiety or nervousness. These feelings help keep us safe and alert us to danger. However, these feelings do not necessarily indicate that danger is imminent. Students should understand, for example, that speaking in front of a group makes most people nervous, but with time and practice, those feelings can decrease.

Stepping outside of our comfort zones and being in situations that bring a bit of discomfort can be good practice for times when these feelings are more intense. Of course, we don't want to put students into situations that cause great anxiety or fear. Taking the previous example, students who are nervous about speaking in front of others should be given the opportunity to do so in controlled situations. Rather than having a very nervous student come up to the front of the class to speak, have them practice speaking with partners, then in triads, then in small groups of four students, and then in a slightly larger group of five or six students, and so on. While the student may feel some discomfort as the groups get larger, you will be providing an opportunity for students to adjust to that discomfort and get through it in a safe and productive way.

Once students are able to better identify their emotions, they will be better able to manage those emotions. It can be especially challenging for students to identify uncomfortable emotions, such as anger, regret, sadness, and anxiety. Children are not necessarily born with the ability to identify their feelings and emotions, especially when they are intense or complex; many teachers have experienced students who lash out when angry, at times behaving violently or aggressively, or shut down when they are frustrated. But students can learn to cope with their emotions in more positive ways once they recognize those feelings and emotions.

You may have heard someone say "use your words" when a child is feeling angry or acting out. This is important, but have we shown students alternative ways to express how they are feeling? Have we shown them how to deal with and clearly yet respectfully express their anger? It is important for us to express our feelings and to model for students how we deal with emotions. For example, we might share that we are frustrated or angry and explain how we deal with the emotion by recognizing that we are angry and expressing that feeling, making good decisions to help resolve any problems or issues, and taking responsibility for our actions. Modeling appropriate courses of action based on our emotions should be explicit.

Once we have begun the process of modeling behavior, we can share ways that

> ## Competency Connections
>
> Self-awareness is a pivotal competency. It leads to self-management, as students must first be aware of and understand their feelings and emotions to manage their emotions and recognize the feelings and emotions of others. When we recognize our feelings and emotions, we can make good decisions about how and when to act on them.

students can practice identifying, expressing, and dealing with uncomfortable feelings themselves. We can share with students a variety of strategies to use when they experience uncomfortable emotions and then have them practice those strategies. It may be helpful to discuss and practice these strategies outside of a time when we are actually experiencing the emotions. In that way, we provide students with opportunities to practice when the stakes are low and when they are not trying to manage challenging or uncomfortable emotions. Then when they do experience those emotions, they will be better equipped to implement the strategies, because they already have some familiarity with them.

 ## Using I Statements

The language people use matters; specificity about what caused an uncomfortable feeling is important. When students are learning to identify the causes of emotions, such as triggers, it is important that they identify their reactions first, rather than point to something outside of them causing the feelings. For example, instead of saying, "That made me mad," students can identify the feelings they had by saying, "When _____ (action, event, etc.), I felt _____." Even more powerful is teaching students to use an *I* statement, such as "I feel _____ when _____." This changes the sense that the emotion was caused by an outside force to the recognition that it was the student's own reaction to something external. This helps students begin to realize that they are not in control of other people's actions or emotions. Their actions affect other people, and their reactions and emotions are up to them.

 ## Emotional Thermometers

Emotional thermometers are tools that students can use to identify their emotions and take appropriate actions, as needed. The thermometer lists a scale of emotions and can include actions to be taken at certain "temperatures," or when students experience those emotions. The purpose is twofold—to share with students that there are gradations of emotions and to offer suggestions of actions they might take when they are experiencing those emotions.

To develop an emotional thermometer, begin by engaging students in an "antonym scales" activity. In this activity, students are given two words that represent opposing emotions. For example, you might start with happy/sad, mad/content, or brave/scared. In pairs or small groups, have students discuss the variety of emotions that fit in between their two antonyms. As they discuss the range of emotions that fall between these antonyms, students can rank the intensity of the emotions. Have students in upper grade levels brainstorm words that go beyond the words presented. (This can also be an additional challenge for younger students.) For example, for the happy/sad antonym range, they may add *ecstatic* on one side and *devastated* on the other. Conduct this activity as a whole group first, and then students can provide additional scales in small groups. Once each group has brainstormed a list of words, review the list as a whole class and brainstorm additional words, or adjust the order of words slightly, as desired.

Elementary Level Antonym Scale Example (Brave/Scared)

brave | strong | fearless | fearful | shy | afraid | **scared**

Secondary Level Antonym Scale Example (Happy/Sad)

ecstatic | elated | delighted | cheery | merry | jolly | **happy** | sunny | pleased | content | neutral | dissatisfied | serious | upset | **sad** | down | sorrowful | depressed

Tip!

Using paint chips, have students write in the range of words on the antonym scale, with each word written on a different color on the chip.

Building Students' Mindfulness

Mindfulness has gained attention in schools in recent years, and for good reason. Many teachers have noticed an uptick in students who have shorter attention spans, who lack focus, and who are easily distracted. Mindfulness is the practice of being aware of the present moment, our thoughts, our feelings, and our environment. Essentially, it is self-awareness, social awareness, and the ability to focus on our thoughts and feelings without judgment.

While the roots of mindfulness lie in Buddhist meditation, mindfulness as it is currently practiced in schools was developed, in part, by Jon Kabat-Zinn from the University of Massachusetts Medical School. His Mindfulness-Based Stress Reduction program has been adapted for schools, prisons, hospitals, and other contexts since its inception in 1979, and in recent years, schools and classrooms across the United States have begun to implement mindfulness (The Greater Good Science Center n.d.).

Practicing mindfulness has multiple well-documented physical, social, and psychological benefits. These benefits begin to manifest after a few weeks of practice, according to a 2003 study (Davidson et al.). Consider just some of the benefits that may result when students practice mindfulness on a consistent basis.

Physical Benefits

Several physical benefits can be attributed to mindfulness practice, including a boost in our immune systems and improved sleep quality. Given that the spread of germs can cause students to miss school, a stronger immune system may lead to fewer missed school days and minimize disruptions to learning. Additionally, higher sleep quality may lead to an increase in focus, attention, and readiness to learn.

Mindfulness also changes our brains in positive ways. Studies of the brain in people who practice mindfulness have shown greater volume in the hippocampus, which plays a role in our attention, learning, and memory skills, as well as in the cerebellum, linked to emotional regulation.

Social Benefits

In addition to the physical benefits of mindfulness, numerous social benefits have been documented. The physical changes in our brains that help regulate emotions and attention, memory, and learning skills benefit us socially as well, and these changes can also minimize negative emotions and stress. Some researchers have concluded that mindfulness may help combat depression and prevent relapse for those who have experienced depression (Segal et al. 2010).

Studies also suggest that mindfulness can help students ignore distractions (Bennett and Dorjee 2016; Harpin et al. 2016). Distractibility can be a major issue in the classroom, and it can impact the workplace as well, decreasing productivity. Helping students minimize distractions will benefit their learning as well as their future careers.

Mindfulness also helps students develop empathy. Research suggests that training in mindfulness increases activity in neural networks involved in empathizing with others and may increase the likelihood of helping someone in need. Self-compassion is also boosted through mindfulness practice. These skills help enhance relationships, increase self-regulation, and build self-esteem.

Benefits for Teachers

Students are not the only ones who benefit from practicing mindfulness. In addition to the benefits listed previously that apply to everyone, mindfulness can also help us, as teachers, to react more calmly when students push our buttons; to hear, listen to, and receive student feedback; and to adjust instruction accordingly. Additionally, mindfulness may help reduce burnout. In fact, a study from the University of Wisconsin–Madison found significant benefits to teacher mindfulness practice, including reductions in burnout and increases in self-compassion (Flook et al. 2013).

 ## Moment of Silence

This short, simple activity helps students practice focusing on just one thing: their breathing and the movements associated with it. This brings needed oxygen to the brain. During a Moment of Silence, instruct students to focus their attention on their breathing, taking two to three deep breaths. They should breathe in through their noses and out through their mouths and focus on the movement of their chests as their lungs expand.

Having students stand up during this time provides the brain with additional oxygen and glucose-rich blood that it needs to focus more efficiently and more effectively. If desired, adding some simple stretches can also help students focus and oxygenate their blood.

 ## Mindful Moment

One strategy for helping students focus is the Mindful Moment. Begin by having students look around their environment, either in the classroom or, preferably, outside. Explain that they will be looking for and at something they have not considered before, maybe an item that interests them—something that catches their eyes—or an item that might be of interest to others.

During a set amount of time, have students concentrate on the object, noticing the size, shape, age, origin, material, texture, and so on, as well as emotions that may be evoked through this careful observation. During this time, students sketch or write about the object, using freeform note-taking, including sketching images and jotting words and/or phrases that relate to the object. This activity can be timed or open, and it can be a very short time frame or a slightly longer time frame, depending on the context.

After the observation, encourage students to share their observations and descriptions with partners or in small groups of students. Share with students that they have just begun to attempt to focus completely on an object and to attend to it fully. From here, they will be moving toward attending to themselves more completely, to becoming more aware of how they are feeling in a particular moment.

Share with students that it is easy to get stuck in times and places other than the present. We sometimes dwell on what has happened earlier in the day or week or focus on something in the future (a test, a sport competition, an upcoming event). Next, have students attempt to attend to themselves by first focusing on their breathing. Have students silently attend to their breaths, noticing if they are shallow or deep and how their lungs expand and how their chests move as they breathe in and out. Point out that our breaths are often shallow at this point, which can result in reduced oxygenation of the body. Ask students to now breathe deeply, feeling their bellies expand and contract as they breathe in and exhale all the way.

Debrief the exercise, and discuss the differences in breathing techniques. From here, students can be guided to begin paying attention to their feelings in the given moment, both physically and emotionally. Encourage students to avoid judging

Tip!

Be aware that students who have experienced complex trauma will likely need modifications for mindfulness practices. For some, mindfulness will be a trigger, and they will be unable to participate in a quiet reflection. If you know that certain students have this background, you may want to give them a different task to do either alongside the activity or in another classroom. Always give students the option of doing mindfulness strategies or activities with their eyes open or with their eyes focused on a place on their desk or the floor.

themselves and their ability to pay attention (or not) during this exercise. This attentiveness on a moment-to-moment basis will help build self-awareness skills and ultimately help students regulate their emotions.

Using Metacognition as a Tool

Metacognition is an important yet sometimes underemphasized aspect of self-awareness. Metacognition refers to thinking about our thought processes, monitoring those processes, and taking control of progress in learning. Self-awareness and metacognition are interwoven. When discussing character strengths and personality traits and helping students consider their own behaviors and motivations, we are encouraging them to be metacognitive.

Metacognition has many benefits. For example, John Dunlosky found that "teaching students how to learn is as important as teaching them content, because acquiring both the right learning strategies and background knowledge is important—if not essential—for promoting lifelong learning" (Dunlosky 2013, 12–13). And according to Wang, Haertel, and Walberg (1990), metacognition is a critical predictor of learning performance.

We can help students monitor their thoughts and help them understand that just because a thought arises, it does not define who we are. The thoughts that arise within us may come from our past experiences, input we have received over time from our families and friends, media we have consumed, or elsewhere. But thoughts are not necessarily who we are. Thoughts can and should be noticed and considered as helpful or unhelpful and, from there, either acted on or disregarded. While this process is not easy, it is the beginning of self-awareness.

Building Students' Metacognition

Metacognition can be built in multiple ways. To start, define *metacognition* for students in a way that they can understand. With most students, I explain that *metacognition* is "thinking about our thinking and our own mental processes." With younger students, it can be beneficial to use a metaphor, such as being in the driver's seat or having their brains' controllers in their hands, just as we do when playing video games. A remote control or video game controller acts to control an aspect of something from the outside. In video games, we control the movement of a character in the game. Metacognition allows us to control what is happening in our brains. Using a metaphor such as this helps make the concept more concrete and can motivate students to focus on the skills they need to improve their learning.

After defining metacognition, share some of the benefits and examples of how students can use metacognition to improve their learning. For example, when we are playing a video game, we may need the character to slow down or to speed up, depending on what is happening in the game. Metacognition works in the same way; we may realize we need to slow our reading of a complex passage in a text, or we may need to speed up our writing of notes during a video, a discussion, or during planning to write as many ideas as possible in preparation for a writing activity. Have students brainstorm additional examples of times when being aware of their thinking is beneficial for learning. Write these examples on a sheet of chart paper that can then be referred to and added to throughout the school year.

Tip!

To build deep metacognition with students, purposefully integrate both explicit modeling and teaching of metacognitive skills, as well as student practice opportunities.

Throughout instruction, model the metacognitive process by sharing your thinking with students. Some teachers feel that they need to have all the answers or be confident at all times with the information and skills they are delivering and how they are delivering the instruction. But showing students how you work through a mistake by first recognizing and admitting it, and then correcting it, benefits students as they see how metacognition works. Additionally, let students know that your decision-making process is dynamic and that you are always learning and may change direction at any time based on what is happening.

Another way to help strengthen students' metacognitive skills is to capitalize on their prior knowledge and experiences. Brain research shows that when students have knowledge about or experience with a particular topic or scenario, they are better able to recall and elaborate on the topic and new learning becomes easier (Chiesi, Spilich, and Voss 1979). Linking to students' personal life experiences builds self-awareness, can help students find meaning in content learning, and validates students' lives, cultures, and experiences.

Additionally, students can be taught the following process to monitor their thoughts about other people, specific scenarios, or actions. Use the steps shown in figure 1.4 regularly to have students consider and monitor their thoughts so that they can then reconsider unhelpful thoughts. If the steps are taken only occasionally, students' brains will not be trained to consistently monitor their thoughts on their own and will not notice when their thoughts are helpful or unhelpful.

Figure 1.4. The Metacognition Process

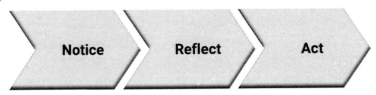

Step 1: Notice

To monitor our thoughts, we have to be aware that they are constantly coming to us and are often fleeting. Students need to know that our thoughts are influenced by multiple factors, including what we see, read, and experience, and by the people who we care about and who are around us. After watching a video clip or commercial, reading a piece of text, or listening to a story, have students write or sketch as many thoughts as they can remember that came up while consuming that media.

Step 2: Reflect

After recording their thoughts, have students categorize them as *helpful* or *unhelpful*. This language is preferable to *positive/negative*, as students should know that a variety of thoughts coming to their minds is a natural and normal part of being human. When we classify the thoughts as helpful or unhelpful, we do not attribute shame to the thoughts that are undesired or unhelpful. Students can annotate the lists of thoughts with a smiling face and an *x,* or with other symbols.

Step 3: Act

Once students have identified thoughts as helpful or unhelpful, they can work to change unhelpful thoughts when they come up. For example, students can make plans or use positive self-talk. Plans may include reframing thoughts, using self-talk to explicitly say that the thought is unhelpful, or saying something such as "I don't really believe that."

 ## Write/Draw It Out

This strategy builds metacognitive skills by having students share what they know about a topic or reflect on their learning through writing or drawing. The purpose is to get students to consider what they know, their background knowledge or past experiences, their learning, and their challenges and successes and apply those to their current or future situations or work. The writing/drawing is built around specific metacognitive prompts you give students, formally or informally. The power of writing/drawing cannot be underscored; it helps students articulate and deepen their thinking about the topic and builds their metacognitive skills.

These reflections can and should be done quickly—they are not meant to be perfect drafts. I find it helpful to give students a specific time frame and then use a timer to keep them accountable to that time. This provides a small amount of pressure and helps keep students on task. As students become more proficient with this strategy (or for older students), you can also add an expectation of the amount of writing or a certain number of items you would like them to add into their writing.

Sentence frames are effective scaffolds and can be used to help students get started. They can be optional or mandatory, but mandatory sentence starters or frames should serve the purpose of increasing students' academic language in writing. Here are sample sentence starters/prompts:

- ▶ The most important part of the reading, video, or class is _____.
- ▶ Two things I know about _____ are _____.
- ▶ How do you feel about this topic? (excited, anxious, curious, nervous, etc.)
- ▶ What do you think of when I say _____?
- ▶ The most useful or valuable thing I learned today was _____.
- ▶ The most surprising or unexpected idea I encountered was _____.

- The ideas that stand out the most in my mind are _____.
- I am most interested in/curious about _____.
- What I know about _____ is _____.
- What helped or hindered my understanding of the reading, video, or class was _____.
- Two ideas that I have found confusing are _____.
- "I learned a lot doing this assignment." I agree (or disagree) with this statement because _____.
- If I were starting this assignment over again, the advice I'd give myself based on what I know now would be _____.
- If I were to paraphrase what we have learned today for a (first-grade) student, it would look like this: _____.
- I am able to connect what I learned today to other topics in this way: _____.

Student Think-Alouds

A think-aloud is when someone (usually the teacher) shares their thinking aloud with others (usually the students). The purpose of a think-aloud is to share the thought process that a skilled person uses. Think-alouds demonstrate self-awareness; one has to be metacognitive and aware of their thought process to engage in a think-aloud. The purpose of Student Think-Alouds is for students to build their metacognitive skills by engaging in their own think-alouds. Model the think-aloud process for students as a means to demonstrate self-awareness. After modeling, have students begin to practice in pairs or small groups. Students can use the sentence frames provided or share their ideas with partners.

Sample Think-Aloud Sentence Frames

Expressing Confusion
- I don't understand _____.
- I was confused when _____.
- I have a question about _____.

Sharing Agreement/Disagreement

- ▸ I agree with _____, and I also think _____.
- ▸ I disagree with _____ because _____.
- ▸ It might be that _____.
- ▸ Another view might be _____.

Discovering New Ideas

- ▸ I just realized that _____.
- ▸ I figured out that _____.
- ▸ What do you think would happen if _____?

Making a Prediction

- ▸ I think that _____ will happen because _____.
- ▸ I don't think _____ will happen because _____.
- ▸ I wonder if _____.
- ▸ Since this happened, what if _____?

Clarifying Something

- ▸ Now I understand _____ because _____.
- ▸ No, I think it means _____.
- ▸ I agree with _____ because _____.
- ▸ At first, I thought _____, but now I think _____ because _____.
- ▸ What I hear you saying is _____.
- ▸ I don't understand _____, but I do understand _____ because _____.

Making a Connection

- ▸ This reminds me of _____.
- ▸ This is like _____ when _____.
- ▸ This is like _____ but is different because _____.

Hypothesizing

- ▸ I (think/predict/hypothesize) _____ will happen because _____.
- ▸ Let's try _____ because then _____.
- ▸ I (think/predict) _____ will occur.
- ▸ Based on _____, I think _____ will happen.

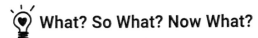 **What? So What? Now What?**

This strategy can be used in several ways. The process is commonly used when reading text or discussing content, and in terms of the metacognitive process, it can be used to help students consider and express what they have learned. The three-step process is fairly simple:

Step 1: What? Students reflect on what they have learned, including new facts, skills, and/or content knowledge that was acquired during the lesson or unit.

Step 2: So What? Students consider the importance of what they have learned, including how the information fits with their background knowledge, how the new information relates to previous learning, and what the information means to them in terms of their long-term goals.

Step 3: Now What? Students consider the next steps. Do they need more information on the topic? What will they do as a result of this learning? What are the next steps that should or need to be taken?

Graphic organizers for the *What? So What? Now What?* strategy can be found in the Digital Resources.

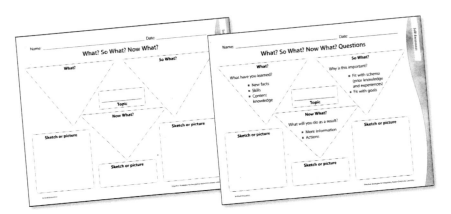

Time and Place

Another aspect of metacognition is to help students determine and understand what helps them learn and that they are likely able to focus more effectively during certain times and in certain places. Have students think about and share when and where they are most able to focus on particular tasks, and ask them to determine why that is the case. For example, students may find that they focus more easily when they are in a brightly lit environment, when it is quiet, or when they have soft music playing. Others may prefer a more dimly lit environment or a place that has more ambient noise. Encourage students to develop self-awareness of when they are most focused and determine the factors that are in place in those scenarios. Note that factors that positively influence focus may change over time, and students should be fluid in their thinking about what helps or hinders their focus and learning. Have students consider the times and places that help them focus several times during the school year. Use these frames as prompts for reflection:

▸ I focus best when _____ because _____.

▸ I focus best in/at _____ because _____.

Stop and Reflect

1. Consider your own level of self-awareness. On a scale from 1 to 5, how aware are you regarding your own identities?

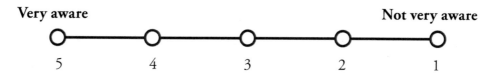

2. On a scale from 1 to 5, how aware are you of your students' identities?

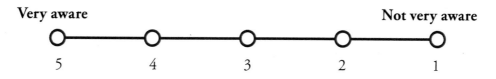

3. How often do you use self-awareness strategies in your own life?

4. Which aspects of self-awareness would students benefit from most in your classroom? Why?

5. What aspects of self-awareness do you already integrate into your instruction? How often do you incorporate self-awareness strategies?

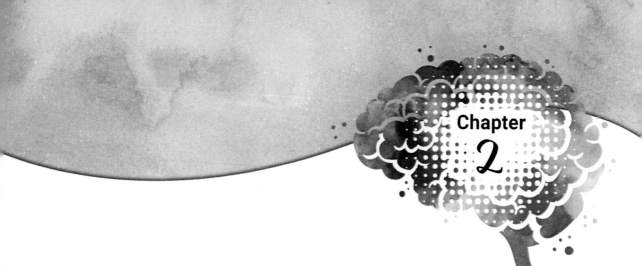

Self-Management

Defining Self-Management

Self-management may be what comes to mind when you consider social-emotional learning, as it includes how students manage their behaviors and emotions in various situations through self-regulation. People with strong self-management skills are able to manage stress using a variety of strategies, self-motivate and take initiative, and use planning skills. Self-management is a critical skill to be successful throughout life.

Mitchem, Young, West, and Benyo (2001) defined self-management as strategies used to alter behavior, frequently to make it less aversive to others and to replace it with behavior that is likely to be more productive. It is the ability to manage your own emotions and behavior given the specific situation. Self-management includes several subskills, including self-monitoring, self-evaluation, and self-reinforcement. These skills are intertwined and enable students to self-manage based on their actual behaviors and the situations or contexts they find themselves in, inside and outside the classroom.

The Importance of Self-Management

Studies show that self-management strategies have helped students improve academic outcomes, acquire and develop social skills, increase on-task behavior, and improve attitudes (Moos and Ringdal 2012). One longitudinal study linked strong self-management skills in children ages 4 to 11 with positive outcomes later in life, including completion of high school and college, financial stability in adulthood, stronger parenting skills, and overall higher life satisfaction. Weaker self-management skills were correlated with negative outcomes, including criminal involvement and drug and alcohol abuse (Knudsen et al. 2006; Moffitt et al. 2011).

Research also tells us that students with self-management skills are better equipped for success and develop better academic skills over time (McClelland et al. 2007). We know that students do better in school when they are able to persevere in the face of challenging content, delay gratification, and focus for extended periods of time. These skills also benefit students later in life as they pursue college degrees or move into their careers.

Impulse control is another key aspect of self-management. While impulse control is somewhat dependent on students' developmental levels, students with poor impulse control face several long-term dangers and problems, and not just in school. Children with low self-control are more likely to be aggressive (Ellis, Weiss, and Lochman 2009; Raaijmakers et al. 2008), to experience depression and anxiety (Eisenberg, Spinrad, and Eggum 2010; Martel et al. 2007), and to commit crimes (Moffit et al. 2011). In addition, there are negative health benefits, including a higher likelihood of obesity, dependency on alcohol and drugs, a higher likelihood of becoming a smoker (Moffitt et al. 2011; Sutin et al. 2011), and suffering shorter life spans (Kern et al. 2009).

In addition, students will face challenging situations in their lives that will require self-management. They may find themselves in situations in which their own identities, norms, or beliefs are questioned, challenged, or even discriminated against. They will likely encounter some tasks they do not want to do or work with someone they do not get along with. Self-managing does not mean that they have to accept injustices or do something they feel is wrong. Rather, it means that in the moment, they may need to manage their feelings and emotions to get through the situation before advocating for or creating change.

Consider the various aspects of identity (e.g., ethnicity, gender, race, nationality, sexual orientation, age, disability/ability, religion, and socioeconomic status). Some aspects of our identity may influence how we handle specific situations and how we choose to self-manage. For example, religious people may turn to prayer, people with wealth may choose to go to spas, and some may choose to take walks through their local parks.

Similarly during class, students will find different ways of self-managing, which may or may not be seen as acceptable to the teacher. For example, an anxious student may self-manage by fidgeting with a pencil or other object, tapping a foot or tapping hands on the desk, or even being disruptive and distracting other students.

Our values and beliefs may impact how we react to a student in these instances. When we see a student who is using a technique to self-manage, we may perceive that the student is taking a needed quick break, or we may believe the student is lazy and disengaged. We might feel that the student should have taken a break during a different time of the day and that this is not the time for that specific action. Our actions can then either encourage or discourage a student's self-management in class.

> Disparaging remarks related to their identities, even if subtle, may cause students to become angry, frustrated, or hurt. Be aware of students' identities, and note when they are self-managing in response to remarks, content, or actions they deem offensive. Address these incidents with students.

Teaching Self-Management Skills

Teaching self-management includes using and sharing strategies that affect student behavior and can positively influence a child's experience. These strategies include the following:

- ▶ Proactive strategies
- ▶ Cognitive strategies
- ▶ Impulse control
- ▶ Self-talk
- ▶ Self-regulation

Teaching self-management strategies to students includes having them consider their goals for the future, think about the best ways for them to avoid or approach specific situations, and practice taking those actions proactively, before the need arises. This is a critical life skill that can be explicitly taught by discussing different scenarios that students may encounter.

Teachers can offer students alternative strategies rather than telling them to stop or to focus, which has been common practice in many classes. Consider the following scenario:

> The teacher is teaching a lesson and including a variety of activities to help keep students engaged and on task. During the modeling and demonstration portion of the lesson, students are engaged and following along, participating in the instruction. After this portion, the teacher moves to having students practice the skills and concepts in small groups. During this practice time, many students are engaged, but there is one small group that is distracted and not working consistently. The teacher walks over to the group and gives them a verbal warning. After checking in with a few other groups, the teacher notices that the group is still off task. The teacher then delivers a consequence to the off-task group, reminding the students that they need to stay focused or future consequences will be more severe.

While off-task behavior certainly needs to be addressed, a potentially more effective way to handle the situation is to teach students how to manage themselves and their behaviors. It may have been that students in the off-task group were not clear about the expectations of the activity. Or they may not have been proficient enough in the skills being practiced. Another possibility is that they may have perceived that they had a low likelihood of success with the task, so they chose not to try. Without self-management skills, students will likely resort to off-task or potentially disruptive behaviors.

Proactive Strategies

Perhaps the first and most important self-management strategies are proactive. Self-management begins with self-monitoring, or considering how we behave in specific situations. Through self-monitoring, students are taught to observe and keep track of their own behaviors. This connection to self-awareness allows students to then take action based on their observations of how they and others behave in specific situations.

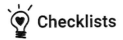

Checklists

One way to help students be proactive in their self-management skills is to help them monitor their actions or the actions of others. Checklists are effective tools for helping students determine what they need to do throughout the day. What may seem obvious to teachers is sometimes mysterious or easy to forget for students. For example, do students know and consider whether they are ready for class with a pencil, paper, and their homework easily accessible so that it can be turned in?

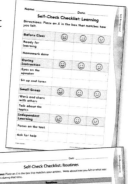

Students should help create these checklists. As students develop deeper awareness of their self-management strengths and areas of need, a checklist can be a useful tool. See the Digital Resources for sample checklists.

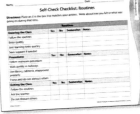

Pre-thinking

Students can also begin to self-manage by considering events and activities— the expectations, what may or may not happen in the scenarios, and how they will respond in various scenarios. This takes a level of experience and maturity that some students may not yet have, but teachers can guide students through it. Explicitly state or ask students to brainstorm the expected behaviors and the likelihood of specific scenarios or actions within a given event. Just as with the checklists strategy, this will help students learn what is expected of them when class starts, during instruction, or when in different areas of the school (playground, lunchroom, and so on).

In the classroom, for example, students can consider how to avoid situations that they know will cause them problems or anxiety. If avoiding the situation is not possible, we need to help students learn how to change the situation or change their actions within that situation. For example, if they know that they are tempted to chat when they sit next to friends in class, they can choose to sit in another part of the room where they will be less distracted.

Literature, current events, and content-related topics can provide excellent examples of pre-thinking self-management skills. As students read books and novels, guide them to consider the characters' actions and self-management opportunities. Similarly, current events can be used to discuss people's actions and self-management, as appropriate. In this way, you can help students pre-think what they might do in different situations. This can also lead to discussions of students' responses to injustices they witness in their communities, the country, and the world.

Pre-thinking Question Examples

- ▶ What will you do in that situation?
- ▶ What are the likely outcomes of your (or others') actions?
- ▶ How could you have planned ahead?
- ▶ What were the consequences of your actions or inaction?
- ▶ What might you do differently next time?
- ▶ How could you have avoided a problem?

 ## Practice Planning

Practice planning is a tool students can use in class. Help students develop plans for how they will work through a particular task. To begin, share with students your own plan for the instructional time. This can be done by reviewing an agenda or the lesson objectives. If the plan changes through the course of instruction, share your thinking and rationale with students. This will model the planning process and the dynamic nature of working through the day.

Students can then practice making plans for how they will tackle a given task. For example, ask students to plan how to get their homework done and turned in on time. For some students, this is a simple task. Others need to consider many things: the time of day they will do their homework, finding a quiet place to do it, where they will keep the homework they need to turn in, and how they will turn it in. Have students discuss their plans in pairs or small groups. Ideas may include putting homework in their backpacks, putting it near their beds so that they see it when they wake up, or putting it near the door.

Cognitive Strategies

Cognition is the process of learning, knowing, and understanding something. Cognitive strategies for self-management involve manipulating our focus or attention in some way, such as through breathing techniques or changing perspectives. Depending on the individual and the situation, one or more strategies may be used. Each strategy can be taught to students and practiced in a variety of scenarios and situations. After teaching the strategies, periodically remind students of the cognitive strategies they can use to self-regulate throughout the day.

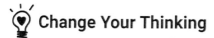 Breathe Deeply

Deep breathing calms our brains, increases our focus, and helps us relax. When something is causing frustration, when more attention to something is needed, or when we feel intense emotions beginning to emerge, deep, slow breaths can help us calm down and manage our emotional state.

> ▸ **Three Deep Breaths (3DB):** Students sit or stand comfortably and as relaxed as possible. They then take three slow, deep breaths. Each breath should be felt not only in their lungs but in their stomachs. Having students put their hands on their bellies can help bring awareness to the depth of their breaths.

> ▸ **Apps and GIFs:** Many apps are available to remind us to breathe deeply, and you may wish to use these apps with students, if appropriate. In addition, you can find GIFs online that encourage students to breathe with the movement of the image.

Change Your Thinking

When students are faced with something they don't want to do, such as a chore, homework, or other activity, help them learn to think about the satisfaction of getting it done rather than focusing on it being something they dread doing. Students can begin to use their thought processes to make the long-term goal more appealing and the distraction less appealing.

Impulse Control

Students can practice self-management by recognizing how and when their distractions, impulses, feelings, thoughts, or actions get in the way of learning and attempting to circumvent them. The goal is to build independence in students so that they can learn to manage their emotions and their actions without direction.

You can support students in developing impulse control in many ways. With all of them, consistency is important. First, begin by giving students reminders about your expectations, pointing out what might distract them during an activity and what they might do to avoid the distraction. Being explicit will help students keep the expectations of an activity in mind and will increase the likelihood of them resisting the impulses (Barker and Munakata 2015).

Along with reminders, use positive reinforcement as students practice impulse control and self-regulation. One issue is students' expectations of a reward for delaying gratification or suppressing an impulse. Some students have been let down or disappointed by promises of a reward or future gratification that never comes. Just a few disappointments will cause a loss of trust and undermine willingness to delay gratification (Kidd, Palmeri, and Aslen 2011). Positive reinforcement can come in many forms and may include pointing out what happens when students control their impulses. Having a discussion, analyzing the process, and supporting students as they work through something can also have a positive impact.

It is also important to consider your reactions to students' emotions when they are both successful and unsuccessful at controlling their impulses. Being dismissive of student emotions by saying things such as "Why would you be sad or angry about that?" or "Calm down!" or "Stop crying!" does not help students regulate themselves or recognize that their emotions are valid. Rather, use phrases that validate students' feelings while providing them the opportunity to self-manage, such as "I can see you are sad; what do you need in this moment? Do you need to talk about it? Or do you need space to be by yourself for a few minutes?" By serving as an "emotion coach," we can help students discuss their emotions and share ways to help them manage their emotions constructively.

Games and role-playing are effective tools for practicing impulse control. Because games are light and playful, they help students learn in a fun and nonthreatening way. These lessons can then be transferred to other areas of life in which self-regulation will be beneficial. The following games can be played in different settings and are fun to integrate when students need a break or when you have a few extra minutes.

Red Light!

One game to help students resist impulses is the traditional Red Light–Green Light game. This game helps students follow directions. But when you add a twist to the game, it helps students go against their impulses and habits. After a few rounds of playing the game, switch it so that *red light* means "go" and *green light* means "stop." After playing the game, point out the skill that students were practicing—going against their first impulses and needing to think carefully before acting.

Move It, Move It

Play music with different tempos. Students dance or move quickly when the tempo is fast and dance or move slowly when the tempo is slow. After a few rounds, switch the directions! This time, students should move slowly during the fast-tempo music and quickly during the slow-tempo music. Point out to students that they sometimes need to be deliberate in their actions and change their behaviors when it does not feel natural.

Memory Games

Research indicates that short-term memory lightens the cognitive load of the frontal cortex of the brain, thereby allowing us to manage impulsivity more effectively (Tarullo, Obradović, and Gunnar 2009). Here are some ideas for memory games:

- **Rhythm Add-On:** Start with a simple clap or movement, which students repeat. Then add one rhythm or movement to the previous rhythm/movement, which the students have to repeat. The back-and-forth continues until students cannot maintain accuracy.
- **Picture Match:** This is a traditional memory game, where students have a set of cards facedown and they have to turn over two cards at a time to find a match. When they match two cards, they collect the pair. The person with the most card pairs at the end wins the round.
- **Vocabulary Match:** This variation of a traditional memory game has students match a word and its correct definition. The player with the most matches at the end wins the round.

Self-Talk

Self-talk is another important aspect of self-management. Research from the University of Toronto (2010) found that using the "inner voice" plays an important role in controlling impulsive behavior. Consider your own actions; you likely have used self-talk to get through a challenging task by setting a short-term goal, reminding yourself of the importance of the task, or thinking through the time line of necessary tasks. Or you may have used self-talk to discourage yourself from eating another cookie or piece of cake, encourage yourself to get to the gym when you felt tired, or prevent yourself from saying something you shouldn't to a friend.

This research has important implications for students; we need to not only teach them that self-talk is helpful but also teach them what self-talk looks like and how they can use it in class and in their lives.

Self-Talk Directed Draw

This is a simple way to teach self-talk to students. Sample directions are provided here, but you can adjust the steps as appropriate for students.

1. Tell students that self-talk is just as it sounds—telling yourself what you need to do or should do.

2. Tell students to repeat the directions you give to themselves in a quiet voice and then follow those directions. You can have students attempt to draw a specific (but simple) image or a series of shapes. For example:

   - Draw a large rectangle.
   - Draw a line dividing the rectangle in half.
   - Draw a circle on the top of the rectangle.
   - Draw a smiley face in the circle.
   - Draw a star in each section of the rectangle.

3. Have students compare their drawings with one another to determine if they have the same drawings or patterns.

Students should not be discouraged if their drawings don't match, as they were relying on your instructions, which may or may not have been specific. In fact, it can make the exercise more interesting if there are some vague descriptions, such as where exactly to put shapes or the exact sizes. The point of the activity is to model and practice self-talk. This can then be transferred to completing other more challenging tasks.

Pausing

Teaching students to pause and to wait two minutes before acting on an impulse can also be a helpful strategy. For example, if a student wants to get up to throw something away or to ask you a question during an independent task, ask the student to wait two minutes. The impulse may wane during that time, or their question may get answered. For younger students, two minutes may be too long, so adjust the time to 90 seconds or one minute, as appropriate. Having an analog clock on display or using a timer can help students track their wait time.

Self-Regulation

Self-regulation is an important aspect of self-managing; it is the biological component. Teaching self-regulation includes teaching students about our biology and how a "system override" can happen when things are not going as planned. In other words, we can have an involuntary reaction to everyday experiences, and this reaction is based on biological functioning, not on our personality or on aspects we can control.

Our daily routines and expectations play into our ability to regulate, starting with our routines when we get out of bed in the morning until we go back to bed at night. During the course of the day, we are getting feedback to and from our biological systems about whether things are OK. When things go well and as planned, our biological systems feel calm. However, if some things go awry, we feel on edge.

> The limbic system is a group of seven brain structures that are involved in processing and regulating emotions and memory, among other things (Okun et al. 2004). It is an important element of the body's response to stress and is highly connected to the endocrine and autonomic nervous systems.

You've probably had students who were easily upset or who exploded for seemingly no reason at all. These are examples of students who have constantly overactive limbic systems, likely because of adverse childhood experiences. In other words, they are reacting involuntarily to things in the environments that have pushed their biological capacity to manage themselves. Learning is overridden by their biology.

For learning to occur, students' limbic systems should not be active. In this biological state, students' brains are primed for learning. This is easier said than done, because each child has diverse background experiences, out of our control. But we can do our best to provide safe and predictable classes with routines and structure, while building on our relationships with students.

Every person reaches moments of frustration where they may have an outburst. During class, these can be disruptive to learning and to the environment. One student's outburst can have a negative effect on the whole class, including on us as teachers. However, these outbursts are the perfect opportunity to point out, teach, and practice self-management and self-regulation skills.

This biological process can be taught to students (even the youngest students) in many ways. You might begin with primary-level students by having them point to their heads or touch their heads and explain that our brains are inside our heads. Explain that the brain is responsible for many aspects of our daily lives, from the five senses to our emotions and memories. Show older students a diagram of the brain and point out the various parts that make up the limbic system. This does not have to be an in-depth science lesson; rather, it should be an introduction to how the brain works and how it relates to self-regulation.

"Flipping Your Lid"

Dan Siegel (2010) explains the process of the limbic system being activated as "flipping your lid" and uses a hand model to demonstrate this to students. In this model, your forearm is considered the spinal cord, and the bottom of your palm is your brain stem. The thumb represents the limbic regions: hippocampus and amygdala. If you tuck your thumb into your palm and fold your fingers over the top of it, you have a physical representation of the brain. In this model, lifting the fingers exposes the limbic system, and this is referred to as *flipping your lid*. When your lid is flipped, your cortex is offline and you have to work on calming down. We want the cortex folded over for full brain function and for learning to occur. It's a practical way for students to understand this biological process.

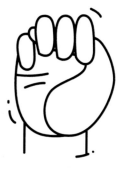

Your Brain

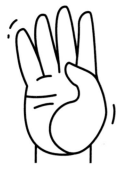

Flipped Lid

 ## All Shook Up

For younger students, use a glitter jar to demonstrate the effects of this biological override. Fill a jar with water and add a few tablespoons of glitter. Tighten the lid so that the jar is sealed. Then shake the glitter jar to show how your brain feels when you are overwhelmed. The glitter settling at the bottom of the jar represents our bodies feeling calm and our brains functioning in a more manageable way.

 ## The Vacation Station

Students may need short breaks throughout the school day when they become frustrated, upset, distracted, or are getting tired. The Vacation Station, the Calming Corner, or the Take-a-Break Space is a designated area of the room where students can go to take a short "vacation" or break. It is important to help students manage these breaks, as they may want to use the breaks as distractions rather than as a useful tool to help manage emotions.

To develop a Vacation Station:

▸ Designate a place in the room where students can cool down or take a short break when they feel triggered, upset, or fatigued. This should be a place where they will not distract or be distracted by others.

▸ Equip the space with a few essential tools, which can be modified, added to, or adjusted based on the time of year, the student population, and students' experiences with using the station. Potential tools may include those listed on the following page.

- ❏ **Primary Level:** stuffed animals, picture books, crayons and paper, and a small timer
- ❏ **Intermediate Level:** All the primary-level items, plus fidget toys, modeling clay, or squeeze balls. Note that these are tools, not toys. The idea is that students have something to hold or use to distract themselves as they process their feelings.
- ❏ **Middle and High School Levels:** fidget toys, modeling clay, squeeze balls, liquid motion bubblers, paper and pens, graphic organizers, markers, magazines, books and short stories, and a timer

Paper and pens or pencils are critical tools for the Vacation Station. Writing, sketching, or doodling is a great way for students to process their feelings and thoughts. Primary students might draw what is happening or how they are feeling. Intermediate-level students as well as older students might write about their feelings, what is happening, or goals to rectify the situation. Some students have reported that writing their feelings, especially when angry, frustrated, or upset, and then crumpling or tearing their papers and throwing them away was a helpful way to release their feelings.

Similarly, reading can be used as a calming tool for students. Consider keeping copies of their favorite books at the Vacation Station. In the Digital Resources, there is a list of books in which the characters demonstrate self-management.

Providing students with additional calming strategies while they are at the Vacation Station gives them opportunities to try other ways to self-regulate. Strategy cards can be printed and laminated. See the Digital Resources for printable Calm-Down Cards.

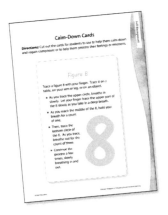 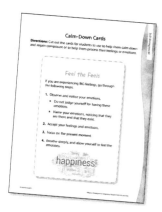

The final and perhaps most important tool is a timing device. Students should know that their time here is valuable and limited. I do not recommend strictly enforcing timing; however, it can be used to give students the opportunity to check in with you. For example, you might include a timer that is set for three minutes. After three minutes, students can either rejoin the class or check in with you and share that additional time is needed. After the second round, you may choose to have a deeper conversation with the student or seek additional support from the school counselor if the student is unable to rejoin the class. A small sand timer such as those found in board games works well.

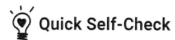 ## Quick Self-Check

In a quick self-check, the teacher pauses and asks students to consider their levels of engagement or focus during whole-class, small-group, or individual activities. It is important to build in checkpoints strategically. In other words, self-checks should not be used only out of frustration when you see that students are off task. This would make the activity more of a punishment than a reflection. At regular, planned intervals throughout a day or week, have students consider their levels of engagement.

To implement this strategy, begin by planning questions that tie in to self-awareness. Sample questions include the following:

- Were you engaged during the last activity?
- What led to your level of engagement?
- What made the activity interesting or engaging to you?
- When did you notice you were off task?
- How did you feel when you began to be disengaged?
- What strategies might help you stay engaged?
- What could you have done differently?
- What could I (the teacher) have done differently?

A rubric may also be helpful in the reflection process. Giving students a simple scale to reflect on can help them more accurately describe their levels of engagement and consider how they can self-manage to be more engaged and focused. The following examples can be modified or adjusted to meet your needs.

Self-Check for Younger Students

4	3	2	1

Self-Check for Older Students

4	3	2	1
I was completely engaged and focused on the task or activity. When I became distracted, I noticed right away and actively removed the distraction.	I was engaged the majority of the time. I participated most of the time, with one or two instances of being disengaged.	I was engaged at times but not engaged or participating for the majority of the time.	Little to no engagement. I was off task and not participating in the learning or activity.

Once students have done the self-check, they should write or discuss their reflections. A quick conversation with partners or quick-writes can help students articulate their reflections. While this may not come easily at first, with practice students will improve identifying their levels of engagement at differing times of the day. Later, they can identify what led them to that level of engagement and use this information to create SMART (specific, measurable, achievable, relevant, and time-bound) goals based on their reflections. The goals might be related to eliminating distractions, identifying times when they are off task and actively working on ways to get back on track, or using or finding activities to get focused.

Whole-Class Self-Regulation Strategies

While it may seem counterintuitive that you can help students self-manage by leading the entire class through an activity, you can show students strategies that they can use independently or during class. One key to whole-class instruction is effective modeling. Begin by sharing with students that you have planned some self-management strategies, such as providing times when they can get up and move. Share that self-management is not only effective for in-the-moment situations when we need to do something differently. Rather, we can plan ahead and have some strategies that can be used at any time when we feel like we need a break.

When teaching the following strategies, model them for students as you would any instruction. Share the purpose, which is to build self-management and self-regulation, and then lead students through the strategy.

Body and Brain Breaks

Many teachers are familiar with the concept of brain breaks, especially since the explosion of the "Baby Shark" challenge. "Baby Shark" is a short song/chant that students sing or perform with movements. The idea behind this movement, and any brain break, is to get students up and moving and to take a quick break from the hard work of learning. While "Baby Shark" is one example of a brain break, many others incorporate movement and are fun, engaging, and motivating.

By singing a song or chant, students are switching modalities, and by having students stand up and move, they get the opportunity to oxygenate the brain. If the song is one they know and have been singing repeatedly, the cognitive demand will be low, which helps make the activity more of a brain break. If you use songs and chants that contain vocabulary or unit concepts and information, you will also be subtly reinforcing the key content concepts and vocabulary.

Stretching can also be an effective way for students to release tension, relax, and de-escalate. By taking a short break and leading students through a series of stretching exercises, you are helping students take a brain break and showing them an effective and quick way to self-regulate.

- **Fan Your Hands:** Stretch your arms out in front of you, and spread your fingers as far apart as possible. Relax your shoulders. Breathe in and out at least twice.
- **Wing It:** Sit up or stand up straight with your fingers interlocked behind your head and your elbows out. Keep your shoulders down, lift your chest, and bring your elbows back as far as you can.
- **Reach for the Sky:** Raise your arms with your fingers interlocked over your head. Reach as high as you can.

- **Listen to Your Body:** Lower your ear to your shoulder on one side. Breathe in and out at least twice. Repeat for the other side.
- **Knee Pull:** While seated, bring one knee up to your chest and hold. Breathe in and out at least twice. Repeat for your other knee.

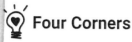

Four Corners

The Four Corners strategy is designed to get students up and moving to a specific area of the classroom. Once there, students engage in a conversation or do an activity. You can get students to the corners of the classroom in a number of ways. You can assign students to a specific corner (numbering off, assigning letters or colors, etc.), or have students choose which area they will go to. For example, in each corner, you can post activities students might like to engage in. Have them go to the corner that fits them best, such as reading, sports, video games, or family time. This activity provides an opportunity to get up and move and can serve as a brain break if the activity done in the corners has lower cognitive demand than the learning students were engaged in prior to moving to the corners.

> ### Competency Connections
>
> Having students work with their peers in a variety of contexts helps build relationships among classmates. Using strategies that build interaction opportunities encourages students to learn more about others, their perspectives, and their ways of thinking.

Find the Match

In this activity, students find a match based on criteria you give them. This strategy uses a physical object such as a sheet of paper with a word, definition, or picture printed on it. You distribute the cards randomly so that each student has a card that matches one or two other cards. Make sure to tell students whether they will match with only one other person or will be forming groups of three. They should be prepared to explain why the words, definitions, and pictures match. As an alternative, take a picture book that is familiar to students. Copy the pages, and cut the text and pictures apart. Hand out the text sections to some students and the pictures to others. Students have to walk around to find the match and explain why the two or three are a match. As an added dimension, play music as students walk around finding their matches.

Stop and Reflect

1. Reflect on your self-management when times are difficult. What strategies do you use, both when teaching and in your personal life, to help you self-manage and self-regulate?

2. How can you make your strategies clear to students so that they see a model of self-management?

3. Consider your vision for students' self-management skills and abilities. What specific strategies will help students attain those skills?

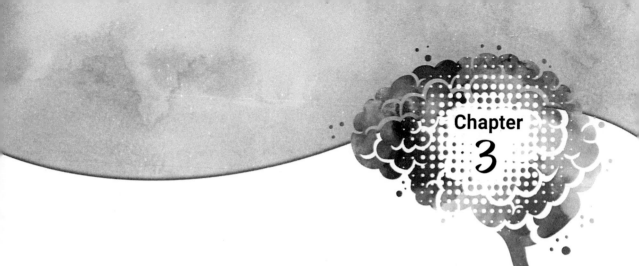

Social Awareness

Defining Social Awareness

Schools are social environments. To be successful in school, students need to recognize and take note of the perspectives of other people, including people from diverse backgrounds and cultures. Therefore, empathy is a key aspect of social awareness. Social awareness also indicates how to behave appropriately in different contexts. Students who are socially aware are able to determine how their own behaviors affect others and are able to do the following:

- ▶ Determine how others feel by analyzing verbal and physical social cues
- ▶ Predict and evaluate others' feelings and reactions
- ▶ Respect others
- ▶ Listen actively to others
- ▶ Appreciate diversity, including individual and group similarities and differences
- ▶ Identify and use family, school, cultural, and community resources

The Role of Emotions

All people inherently know that the feelings of others affect us. As a teacher, your moods and feelings have likely been affected by students in your class. When students are excited or happy about an upcoming event, keenly interested in a story or novel being read, or visibly angry and frustrated about something happening, our moods and emotions can be impacted. While we are professionals who try to not allow feelings of frustration or anger to negatively affect our practice, we cannot completely separate ourselves from our emotions, nor should we.

Students should also be made aware that other people's feelings affect our own feelings. It is clear that humans subconsciously and automatically mimic the emotions of others. For example, if we see someone smiling, we may smile back, or if we see someone frowning, we may also frown. This mimicry triggers reactions in our brains and bodies. Parkinson and Illingworth (2009) found that anger in others, for example, may cause fear about what they are going to do next, cause feelings of guilt about how we may have caused the anger, or cause us to reciprocate the anger. When we perceive the emotions of others, such as anger, we may "reverse engineer" (Hareli and Hess 2010) what caused that emotion and interpret that they are looking for someone to blame and feel that the blame is aimed toward us.

In addition, emotions can be co-constructed and developed based on the interactions one is having with other people (Fogel 1993; Parkinson 2001). Because human interactions are dynamic and relationships play a part in how emotions develop, there is not a simple cause-and-effect relationship between one person's emotions and another person's reactions. Rather, in most instances, there is mutual emotional engagement. Students can and should be asked to consider how their actions and emotions affect others and are affected by others throughout the course of the day.

As a part of teaching self-awareness (Chapter 1), we discussed focusing on helping students name emotions and feelings by teaching them the vocabulary associated with emotions and feelings. Next, they should learn that part of social awareness is recognizing and understanding others' feelings and emotions. This can be done by identifying their own emotions as well as the emotions of others, such as characters in stories, novels, and movies. For younger students, English learners, students with special needs, or students with limited or interrupted formal education, you could begin by giving them labels for emotions, such as sadness, anger, frustration, nervousness, happiness, excitement, or embarrassment. You might use the statements below and show pictures for reference. The following sentence frames can be used to discuss a variety of emotions:

- It looks like they are feeling _____.
- When people _____ (behavior), it might mean that they feel _____. Do you think that is how the character/person is feeling?
- They must be _____ (feeling/emotion) based on what just happened. Is that accurate?
- _____ (situation or behavior) makes me feel _____. How does it make you feel when that happens?
- How do you think _____ feels/felt when _____ happens/happened?

After modeling identifying emotions in characters, you can move on to asking students how characters feel and having them share their responses with partners. These exercises will pave the way for students to discuss their own feelings. Starting this activity early on, with primary-level students for example, will help students who are somewhat reluctant to discuss feelings become more at ease with the topic, especially when it comes time for them to discuss their own feelings.

Some students—including some boys, adolescents, and students from cultural backgrounds and families in which discussing feelings is uncommon—may be hesitant to discuss their feelings with you. By discussing the feelings of others, these students may open up regarding their own feelings over time. This is not to say that students should be required to share feelings publicly, especially when those feelings are uncomfortable. However, students can be provided opportunities to share with you or with another adult, such as a counselor or therapist, if needed.

As students learn to observe how others are feeling in a variety of contexts, they can begin to see how their actions affect others. As needed, check in with students to see what is happening in class and how it makes them, and others, feel. Using "I feel" statements offers students the opportunity to share their emotions in a way that is less confrontational. A classroom culture of respect is required for this, though, as sharing emotions can put students in vulnerable positions, especially when they are feeling angry, sad, or frustrated.

Radio Reading

In Radio Reading, students read specific passages with emotion, based on the events or dialogue in the book or story. Students will need to infer emotions based on actions or descriptions within the text and will likely need instruction to use these context clues. Students then read the text aloud using their voices to exemplify the emotions. Radio Reading is an effective strategy for helping students reread text with a purpose.

 Photo Feelings

People learn to detect emotions in others from a very early age. Early on, we know when our parents or caregivers are upset, calm, or happy, based on their tones of voice, verbal expressions, and physical movements and gestures. This is especially true of more general or extreme emotions. However, children may struggle to discern the more subtle emotions their parents or others may be feeling. As discussed in the self-awareness chapter, learning about feelings and emotions is essentially a vocabulary activity.

Pictures of people expressing emotions can be used for this activity. Begin with pictures that show more obvious emotions. Have students discuss the pictures and explain how they know a particular emotion is being displayed. Use pictures that show a variety of emotions, such as the examples shown here.

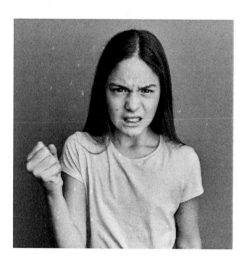 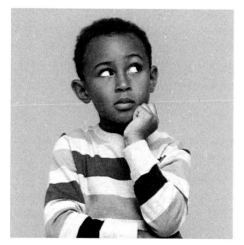

Images of characters from picture books, historical photographs, and other photos can be used to meet students' specific ages, grade levels, and needs.

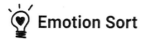 Emotion Sort

Once students are familiar with identifying emotions in photographs or pictures, they can take a set of pictures and sort them on a continuum of emotions. Using a variety of feeling words, students can sort and label the pictures and use the images to brainstorm additional words to describe each emotion on the continuum. By describing the emotions they see in the pictures and discussing the emotions that others might have, they will recognize these emotions in their everyday lives more easily.

Thoughts and Words

In this strategy, students use speech bubbles and thought bubbles to share information about the thoughts and feelings shown in a picture or photograph. Students consider the actions of a person or character (from a story, event in history, etc.) and create speech bubbles showing what was said and thought bubbles showing what might have been going through the person's mind. Alternatively, students can practice this for scenarios you share. For example, students could write what they would say in a given situation and what they might be thinking. This activity can help them gain empathy by considering what people say and do not say in different situations. Here are example scenarios:

- You and your friend are playing with toys that belong to your friend. You really want to play with one of the toys, but your friend won't let you and gets upset when you start playing with a toy when they aren't looking.

- A friend is angry with you. They blame you for something that happened, even though you did not cause the situation. They begin shouting at you.

- A friend tells you that another friend is angry with you because of something you did. When you try to explain to them that you did not mean to upset them, they do not believe you and begin to raise their voice.

- A friend is very excited about an upcoming trip their family will be taking. They want to share the news with you and celebrate.

> ### Competency Connections
>
> Understanding how words affect others builds social awareness as well as self-awareness. When we think before we speak and consider the effect our words might have, we self-manage. Being considerate of others and taking action when we see that something upset someone also develops our relationship skills.

Silent Situations

Another visual strategy for helping students identify emotions is a silent video. Any video clip can become a silent video—just mute the sound. Show students short video clips that include both exaggerated and subtle emotional cues. As students watch the clips, have them identify the emotions displayed and the potential cause of each emotion. For some scenes, the causes may be obvious, but for others, the causes will be unknown, especially if they are verbal.

Real-World Feelings and Emotions

Once students have practiced identifying emotions through visual means, such as pictures and videos, they can explore identifying emotions in others. Using the Real-World Feelings and Emotions strategy, students will analyze literary characters, historical people, and people in their lives. Students can consider how people feel or felt as they read a story, novel, or historical event. As students consider the emotions of the people they are learning about, they can also consider what caused those feelings. Students can make observation journals in which they observe people in their lives and write the emotions they observe. The idea is not for students to identify specific people and their emotions but to reflect on the emotions they see, determine the context of the emotions, and describe how people displayed those emotions.

Guess My Feeling

In this game, students work with partners to show and then identify specific feelings through displaying facial features. There are several versions of this game, depending on students' grade level and maturity.

One version includes having students get into pairs and identify who will be partner A and who will be partner B. Once students are in their pairs, display a feeling word card or a picture card on the board so that only one of the students in each pair can see the card. This may look like having students stand in two rows, with all A partners facing one side of the room and all B partners facing the opposite side. Then display the word to the A partners. Have all A partners make facial expressions to demonstrate that feeling. The B partners must then guess the feeling or emotion being displayed. If you want to keep score, they can earn a point if they guess correctly. Then have pairs switch so that the B partners have a chance to make the facial expressions and their partners get to identify the feelings.

Alternatively, provide students with paper bags or baskets with feeling and emotion word cards or pictures inside. One partner pulls a card out of the bag, looks at the word or picture, and then displays the word or picture through facial expressions. The other partner must guess the emotion being displayed. (See Chapter 1 for a list of feeling words for different grade ranges.)

This activity can also be done as a whole class. Choose one student to come to the front of the room. Have the student sit or stand facing the class. Then show a word card or a picture of an emotion or feeling to the class. The class gives clues about the emotion or feeling to the student in the front. They can use synonyms or describe scenarios or stories to give clues to the person who is guessing. Once the student has correctly identified the feeling or emotion, another student takes a turn.

 Family Feud: Feelings Edition

To play Family Feud, split the class into several teams. These teams can be chosen randomly or assigned using any number of criteria to balance boys and girls, academic readiness levels, English proficiency levels, and so on. Once students are in teams, two teams face off, with one student from each team standing up front to answer. The teacher reads a scenario or describes a feeling or emotion. The first team member to ring a bell, clap, or raise a hand to respond and answer correctly gets points. Then that team member goes to the back of the line, and the next student moves to the front. The team that answered correctly stays standing. The other team sits down, and a new team comes up to face the team that scored. Continue playing until each team has had a chance to earn points. See the Digital Resources for sample game cards.

 Tableau of Feelings

A *tableau* is a group of models or motionless figures depicting a scene from a story or from history. Tableaux are commonly used in theater arts and can be incorporated in any content area to help students practice vocabulary. This strategy is similar to having students show feelings or emotions with their faces; however they will use their entire bodies to represent a scene that evokes emotion or to represent the emotion itself.

Explain to students that they will be using their bodies to create tangible representations of concepts, ideas, or quotes. Allow students to create a true tableau based on relatively simple vocabulary words or ideas. For example, you might start with emotions such as happy, sad, angry, bored, or frustrated. From there, you can ask students to show more complex feelings, such as despair, fury, or anxiety.

Begin by putting students into pairs in which one student will be partner A and the other will be partner B. Consider carefully how you will pair students; they should be paired with peers with whom they are comfortable working, as this activity can be awkward for students who are unused to the physical aspect. Students should stand or sit in a neutral position, as relaxed as possible. Have student pairs shake hands or greet each other. Let students know that partner A (or B) will be a respectful sculptor and the other will be the clay. The sculptor will tell and show the clay how they want them positioned to demonstrate the concept. Give partners a few minutes to practice, and then let them know that when you give the signal, the clay should demonstrate the concept. At that time, the sculptors should look around the room and observe the other ways their peers demonstrated the concept. Students should then switch roles so that everyone has a chance to be both the sculptor and the clay.

> **Tip!**
>
> Offer students the option of greeting each other with a wave and verbally explaining directions and demonstrating what they want their partners to do. This respects students who are not comfortable with touch.

The Role of Social Cues

Communication styles and cultural behaviors vary greatly between different groups. A gesture, joke, or one's tone of voice may be considered lighthearted in one group but extremely offensive in another. The way we communicate and pick up on social cues can affect our relationships, the perceptions others have of us, and the perceptions we have of other people. By teaching students this concept and helping them begin to learn about social cues in different cultures, we can build social awareness and foster positive relationship skills with many different people.

You do not need to be an expert in every culture to begin building awareness. In fact, students may be excellent sources of knowledge on the topic, although they may know it implicitly. Start with a simple discussion of students' experiences and knowledge of the topic. From there, you can begin to discuss these concepts in terms of how they play a part in literature, history, or texts the class is reading. Some key topics include the following:

Eye Contact: Cultures vary tremendously on norms for eye contact (in terms of when it is made, how, for how long, and by whom). In some cultures, there is an expectation of nearly constant eye contact, but in other cultures, the level of eye contact can depend on age and positions of power, for example.

Volume and Tone of Voice: How we say things is as important as—and, in some cases, more important than—what we say. A friendly "Hello" to a friend can be soft and quiet or loud and enthusiastic. We can also say it as a sarcastic question: "Hellooooo?!" In some cultures, speaking loudly indicates anger. In others, volume may indicate an attempt to command attention. The pitch used also has different meanings in different cultures.

Touch: How people use or don't use touch is rooted in culture. Consider greetings, for example. A firm handshake can signify confidence, or it can signify aggression, depending on the culture. People in some cultures use a kiss on one or both cheeks to greet someone. Touching a child on the head can be considered a loving gesture, or it can be considered extremely rude, as the head is considered sacred in some cultures.

Proximity: The amount of space between people when standing or sitting is highly cultural. We each have our own sense of how close is too close, but this varies among people from different cultural backgrounds.

Facial Expressions: Much of communication is nonverbal. How and when we smile at others, for example, can convey different messages. Some people may consider a smile from a stranger or passerby to be a friendly greeting, while others may consider it to be overstepping personal boundaries.

Gestures: There are many examples of gestures that have very different connotations based on the culture. The "OK" symbol, for example, may signify approval, zero or nothing, or an offensive swear, depending on the culture. In some cultures, standing with one foot showing the sole of your foot is considered extremely offensive, while in others no meaning is conveyed by such a stance.

Using literature, movies, or other texts, you can point out to students that cues differ among cultures and that social awareness includes learning about other cultures and how people perceive one another. That's not to say that everyone must be an expert in every culture around the world. That would be extremely difficult, if not impossible. But if we ask students to pay attention to actions and cues, as well as other people's reactions to them, we can help them build deeper awareness of themselves and others and ultimately deepen their relationship skills, too.

Social Cues Role-Play

To practice demonstrating social cues, students can participate in a role-play. Provide each student with a card that lists specific communication styles and behaviors. (Sample cards and scenarios can be found in the Digital Resources.) For example, one student may have a card that instructs them to stand close to someone and frequently look them directly in the eye as they speak. Another card may instruct a student to avoid eye contact and maintain a minimum of four or five feet from anyone they are talking to. Then share a scenario with students, such as meeting for the first time, asking to play a game on the playground, or asking a peer what they missed in class when they were absent. Students should not share the cards and the behaviors with one another. Rather, they should take notice of the social cues that are being demonstrated by their classmates. After the interactions, debrief what students noticed and how it made them feel when the behaviors of their classmates varied significantly from their own behaviors.

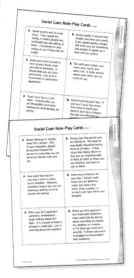

Active Listening

How many times have you said or felt like saying, "If you would have listened…"? Often, we are frustrated by students' (and others') lack of listening skills. Yet many of us do not teach active listening skills to students. Some benefits of active listening are as follows:

- Demonstrates undivided attention to the speaker
- Makes the speaker more likely to continue the conversation and attempt to engage the listener
- Helps restart a stalled conversation or fill in any gaps
- Improves the speaker's insight into the story or issue being discussed
- Reassures the speaker of confidentiality
- Builds rapport

Students can use several observable behaviors to help them listen actively (see figure 3.1). Students should display that they are focused on the speaker; give verbal and nonverbal cues that they are listening; acknowledge the speaker's message; use appropriate linguistic turn-taking; ask clarifying questions; and give an honest, appropriate response. We will explore each of these behaviors and look at some ways students can practice them in the classroom.

Figure 3.1. Observable Behaviors of Active Listeners

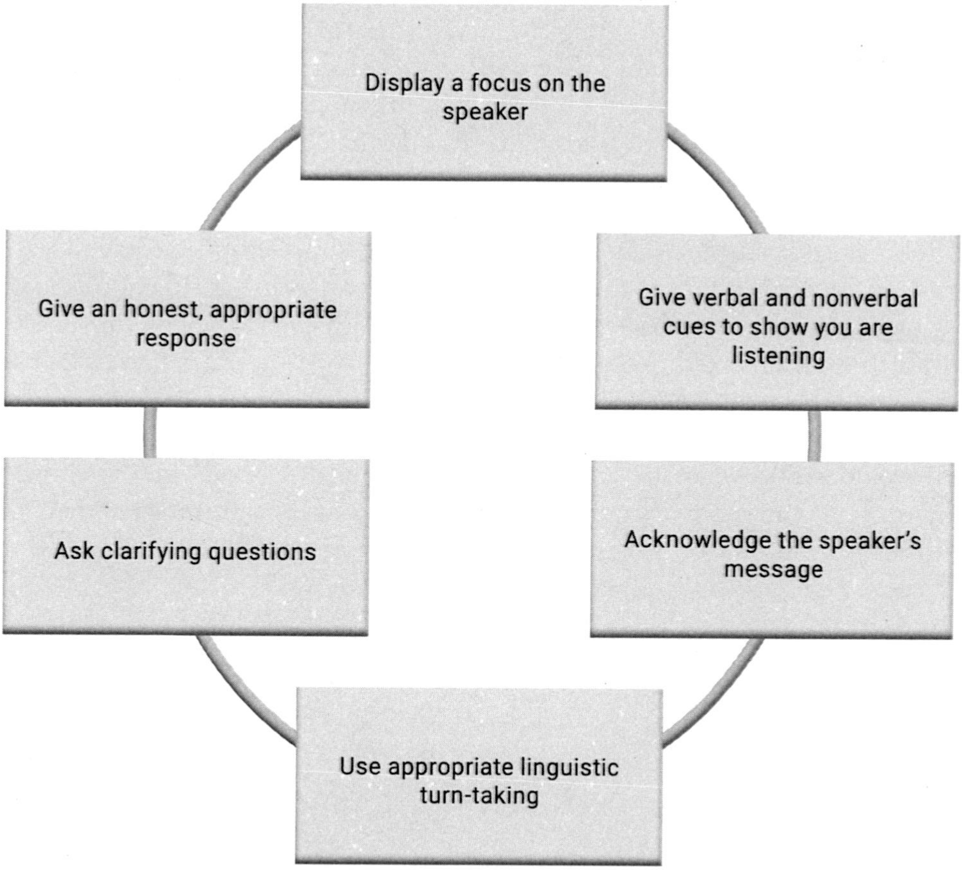

Display a focus on the speaker

Give verbal and nonverbal cues to show you are listening

Acknowledge the speaker's message

Use appropriate linguistic turn-taking

Ask clarifying questions

Give an honest, appropriate response

Display a Focus on the Speaker

First, active listeners indicate that they are listening and focused on the message. This involves looking at the speaker and avoiding distractions, such as looking at other people in the room or looking at objects such as a cell phone or notebook. For some students with special needs and some English learners, appropriate eye contact may need to be taught. Students should not stare at the speaker but should consistently look at the speaker.

Avoiding distractions can be especially difficult for students. However, we can help students practice avoiding distractions by first identifying distractions. If students cannot name them, they will not be able to avoid them. Begin by brainstorming distractions that lead students off task when listening during class. Some ideas include a classmate asking them a question, an unrelated thought that comes to mind, and books or other materials.

After brainstorming and naming some potential distractions, students can learn to track and record instances when they are distracted. What got them off track? How long did it take to get back on track? A simple form can be helpful for you and students to determine additional distractors and the amount of time students can listen without becoming distracted (see figure 3.2). Alternatively, students can use a checklist of the distractors they brainstormed, as well as some you have noticed. They should mark when they notice they are being distracted from attentively listening. It is important that these tools not be used as punishment; they are designed to name and note distractors so that those distractors can be avoided in the future.

Figure 3.2. Sample Form for Identifying Distractions

Date/Time	Student(s)	Distractor	Time Off Task	Helpful Reminders/Notes

Once distractors have been identified and named—and potentially tracked—you can look for patterns to help students to minimize or resist distractions. Provide practice during a listening exercise, a guided practice activity where students work together, or independent practice by asking students to intentionally focus and avoid distractions. Keep these practice opportunities short, based on students' age, maturity, and distractibility. The idea is to help them practice avoiding distractions in a controlled setting and to gradually build up the amount of time that they stay focused.

In essence, when students avoid and minimize distractions, they are listening to understand the message rather than focusing on their own ideas or how they will respond. Students should attempt to remain neutral while listening. Removing or ignoring distractions also helps listeners observe the subtle expressions and movements the speaker is making, which, in turn, will help the listener better understand the message.

Use Verbal and Nonverbal Cues

In addition to avoiding distractions and using eye contact, the next aspect is to use verbal and nonverbal cues to show the speaker that you are listening. These include nodding or otherwise signaling agreement or using other appropriate facial expressions, such as surprise, sadness, or glee. Students should be seated or standing in a position that shows they are listening. For example, students should sit up straight or stand up straight, with their feet flat on the floor and their faces and bodies toward the speaker. Students can be shown example pictures and can then practice appropriate sitting or standing positions. They can also demonstrate inappropriate ways to sit or stand.

Acknowledge the Speaker's Message

Another key aspect of active listening is acknowledging that you have heard the message. Of course, communication is a two-way street; the speaker delivers a message, and the listener receives it. As a part of this process, the listener should acknowledge that the speaker has been heard and that the message was understood. All the aspects discussed thus far will help, but verbalizing what the listener has heard will help the speaker know that the message was received accurately. One way to do this is to repeat what you have heard. Students can share what they have heard in three ways:

- ▸ **Repeat:** The listener essentially repeats the message using the speaker's exact words, as closely as possible. Students may not be able to remember every word, so they will need to listen for key words and incorporate them as they repeat what was said.
- ▸ **Paraphrase:** The listener shares what the speaker said, this time using words that are similar to the ones used by the speaker. The listener summarizes what the speaker has said or shared.
- ▸ **Reflect:** The listener reflects on the message and responds using their own words. The listener summarizes their understanding of the message.

Use Appropriate Linguistic Turn-Taking

Some students are more extroverted than others, some are fast processors of information and are able to respond quickly, and others need more time to think and reflect. In any case, there are certain cultural norms around linguistic turn-taking that students may or may not be consciously aware of. These include noticing and acting on the subtle clues speakers give in a conversation and appropriately commenting on what was said, asking clarifying questions, or extending the conversation by adding information or a comment.

The rules of turn-taking in conversations vary among cultures and take into consideration a variety of factors, including the relationship between the speaker and listener, the power dynamic between the speaker and listener, the ages of the speaker and listener, and the context of the conversation. It is important that students understand these dynamics and learn how to respond appropriately.

To have students practice linguistic turn-taking, consider incorporating multiple protocols that students can follow when having conversations with partners or in small groups. These protocols can be used in isolation or combined to help students practice turn-taking.

 ## Talking Chips

This strategy is best used in small groups. Each student receives a certain number of chips or small objects. To add to the conversation, you must put in a chip. Once you run out of chips, you are no longer able to add to the conversation. When using talking chips, make sure to keep the activity short enough that students are not left out of the conversation for long periods of time.

 ## Talking Stick

This strategy is best used in small groups. Give each group one object, such as a stuffed animal, a wand, or a squishy ball. Each person takes a turn picking up the object and speaking. Only the person who has the object can speak at any given time. After speaking, they put the object down, and the next person picks it up and speaks. To reduce the spread of germs, each student can have an object in front of them, but only one student at a time can hold the item and speak.

 ## All Voices Heard

With this protocol, each student's voice must be heard before anyone can add to the discussion a second time. Because some students may not feel comfortable right away, provide students the option to say "pass" if they do not want to add more. This ensures each student's voice is heard, but students have the option to not speak extensively.

> **Competency Connections**
>
> Active listening is a key relationship skill. As students become better listeners, they may deepen their relationships with others and become more aware of other people's thoughts, motivations, feelings, and emotions.

 ## Timed Talk

Use a timer to indicate the amount of time each student can talk. Each group can use their own timer, or you can set a timer for them. Each student in the group talks for a set amount of time, from just a few seconds to a minute or more, depending on the context. If the student finishes speaking before time is up, the group waits in silence until the person says more or the timer goes off.

Ask Clarifying Questions

Active listeners ask clarifying questions when they do not understand something. One way students can practice this is by first acknowledging the speaker's message, as described previously. Before or after repeating, paraphrasing, or reflecting, the student might add one of the following phrases to make sure the message was understood appropriately:

- "When you said _____, did you mean _____?"
- "I am unclear about _____. Can you tell me more?"
- "Did you mean _____?"
- "I don't quite understand why _____."
- "Can you please repeat the part about _____? I didn't hear/understand what you said."

Of course, students can use many other phrases to ask clarifying questions. The key is to include this practice as needed as part of the active-listening routine.

Give an Honest, Appropriate Response

The last aspect of active listening is to respond appropriately and honestly to the speaker about the message they are sending. This can be challenging for people, as we need to be able to express ourselves in an honest way but also be respectful of the person and their needs. When we respond appropriately and honestly, we take into account the needs of the person, as well as our own needs and feelings. Share the following elements of an honest and appropriate response with students, and have them practice incorporating these elements into their responses.

1. **What does the person want to know or hear?** You should not focus on only telling someone what they want to hear. Rather, focus on what information they are requesting. Would they like your opinion, are they seeking acknowledgment, or are they seeking specific information from you?

2. **How much of a response should I give?** Consider how much you should talk in response to the person. If the person is upset about something or in distress, it may be that you do not need to say much other than to acknowledge what you are hearing, as discussed earlier. If you are discussing ideas for an event such as a birthday party or a vacation, a lengthier response would be appropriate.

3. **What will be helpful to this person in terms of my response?** While we sometimes feel that holding back a part of our reactions and feelings may be dishonest, we should also consider what will actually be helpful. For example, if we have a visceral reaction to something someone said, or vehemently disagree, we can share the parts of our reaction that people can process and not share those aspects that the person might feel are offensive or hurtful.

This aspect of active listening is likely best practiced by you. Young students may not have the maturity level to deeply understand these elements. However, as students move into the secondary level, it may be appropriate to incorporate aspects of these elements into your conversations. For example, you might point out what was not said in a conversation between characters in literature.

Acronyms for Active Listening Skills

Several acronyms can help students incorporate or implement the skills of active listening. Each one focuses on slightly different aspects of active listening and can be used with students to help them deepen their social-awareness skills. Choose the acronym that best fits students' needs and your teaching style. Once students have had the opportunity to practice these skills, you can have them reflect on and write about what it takes to be a good listener.

A poster version of each acronym can be found in the Digital Resources.

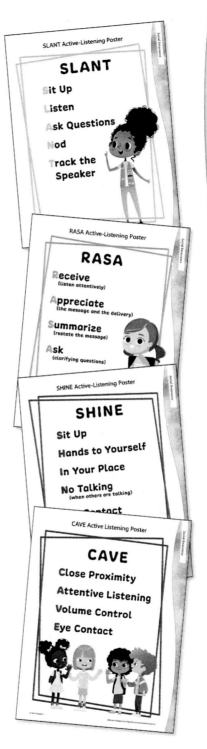

The Reflective Cycle

As students get older and truly become socially aware, they need to reflect. To do this, you can lead students through a reflective process in which they consider the event, their involvement, and how the event affected the people involved (see figure 3.3). The steps that follow demonstrate the reflective process. This process can be used to develop social awareness through reflecting on literature, historical events, and classroom/school events or incidents.

1. **Consider the event.** What is the event you are focusing on, and why are you focusing on this event? In the classroom, we sometimes dissect only a particular event because someone is upset, angry, or hurt. But to help students develop social awareness, we should also consider events that brought up pleasant feelings, such as happiness, joy, and laughter. Students can identify key events in a story, in history, or in their lives for this purpose.

2. **Consider feelings.** How did the character in the story, person/people in history, or you feel before, during, and after the event? How do you know? Consider the emotions displayed before, during, and after the event and what signals were noticed or not noticed about the display of those emotions. You may want to focus on the feelings and emotions vocabulary exercises that were done as part of building self-awareness (see Chapter 1).

3. **Consider the outcomes.** What was the outcome of the event? How did this affect the characters and/or people involved? When considering your own involvement in a particular situation, think about how your feelings and emotions affected the outcome. How did others react based on what they thought you were feeling or emotions they thought you were displaying?

4. **Consider alternatives.** Based on what you have considered thus far, what could or should have been done differently? What should the characters or people have done or not done? How did or could the person have controlled their emotions to affect the event?

5. **Consider/create a different course of action.** Once you have considered the alternatives, create an action plan. What is the desired outcome from here? What are or should be the next steps?

Figure 3.3. The Reflective Cycle Graphic Organizer

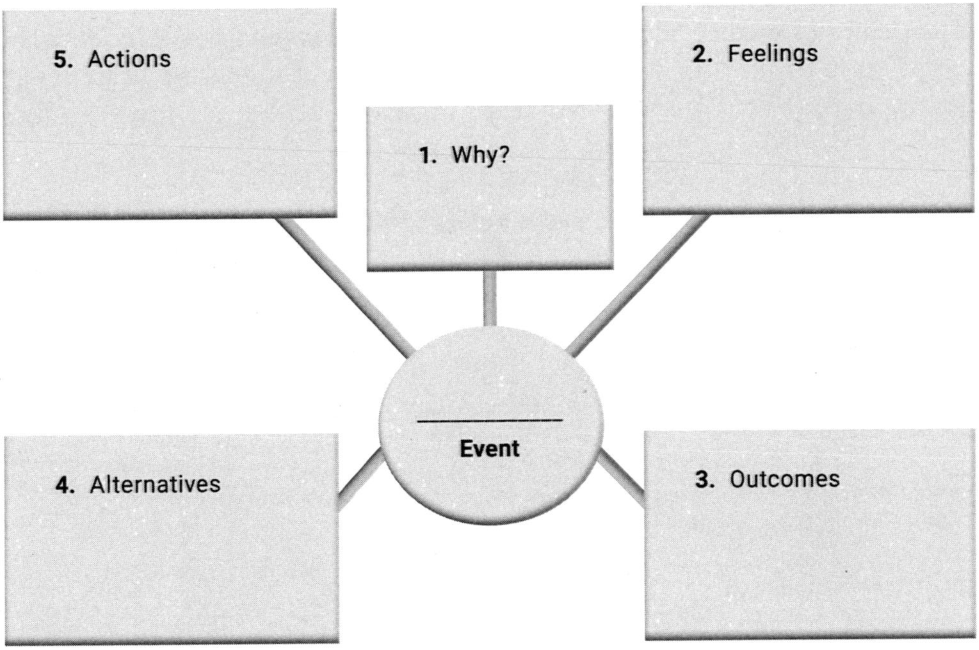

5. Actions	1. Why?	2. Feelings

Event

4. Alternatives		3. Outcomes

The Role of Social Justice

Why do discrimination, prejudice, racism, religious intolerance, and other forms of bigotry exist? In part, it is likely because people fear the unknown. When people are unfamiliar with or do not know about the cultures, traditions, and ways of thinking of others, they experience fear. That fear can then turn into intolerance, bigotry, prejudice, and so on. Sometimes, people are unaware that culture deeply influences how others behave. They may not understand why a person is behaving in a certain way—they may not understand that the intention is not to cause offense or because they are wrong or have bad intentions. Rather, they are following their own patterns of behavior, which are dictated in large part by culture.

Social justice refers to fair and equal treatment of and between individuals in society, regardless of their identities. Social awareness builds social justice. As students learn more about one another and more about people who are culturally different from them, they begin to build understandings of others and different ways of thinking and being.

Students learn very quickly the concept of fairness. As they develop social awareness, they can also learn that some groups are not treated fairly because of their cultures or their identities. Students can and should begin to learn this concept very early in their school careers. The idea is not so much that we should expose very young children to the horrors of society. Rather, students can learn that their actions and values affect others and how they feel about and interact with others. We should be aware of other people and how people are sometimes treated differently than we are. This, in turn, builds respect and empathy as we deepen our social awareness.

Tip!

Build your own awareness of the community you serve by identifying and visiting places of cultural importance to students and families you work with. Survey students and their families about where they shop, recreate, worship, or gather, and visit those places in the community.

Outside and Inside

Sometimes students need a simple lesson to reinforce that we all have identifying characteristics on the outside, but on the inside, we have different characteristics that are hidden. This activity is adapted from a strategy shared in an article by Kassondra Granata (2020) in *Education World*.

1. Give each student a piece of citrus fruit. You can use one type or a variety, but if you are using a variety, make sure to have several pieces of each kind of fruit.

2. Have students study their pieces of fruit, looking for specific defining characteristics. If desired, have them write a few of the defining characteristics. Collect the fruit and put it in a bowl or bag.

3. The next day, have students find their pieces of fruit based on the characteristics they noted. Then have students trade their fruit with another student.

4. Once students have someone else's fruit, have them peel the fruit and put it back into the bowl or bag. Instruct students to now try to find their specific pieces of fruit. It will be essentially impossible, as the outer characteristics have been stripped away.

5. As an alternative, safely cut up the pieces of fruit rather than have students trade fruit and peel it. While this is a bit more time-consuming, by giving students a few wedges of the fruit to taste, they may be able to determine the kind of fruit they had, even though it may not be the exact fruit piece.

6. Debrief the activity by discussing how we often use visible or outside characteristics to identify something or someone, but we need to get to know that person to know what is on the inside.

 ## Stand Up and Be Recognized!

In this activity, the teacher begins by recognizing and making public the actions of students that benefited others or the class as a whole. It will be important that you look for opportunities to recognize each child in the class. As time goes on, students are asked to reflect on the roles their peers played in building success for the class or group with which they were working. This reflection helps students see that their actions and the actions of others contribute to the success of the group. Have students consider how someone in their group or in the class contributed to the success and well-being of others. The student sharing asks that person to stand up and be recognized for their contribution. Identify the various actions, activities, or materials that were used in the lesson and how their actions and involvement contributed to success. Celebrate the person or people being recognized through a round of applause, a class cheer, or by a choral "Thank you!" shared by the class. Have students share or write one or two sentences that explain their choices.

Empathy as a Key Social-Awareness Skill

Empathy is not necessarily an innate human trait. Through our social interactions and relationships, we learn to be empathetic. We appreciate when others show empathy toward us and learn that showing empathy to others strengthens our relationships. As teachers, we focus on teaching empathy, often implicitly, as we encourage students to build strong relationships with one another, teach them to listen to us and to one another, understand verbal and nonverbal cues, and appreciate our differences.

Research shows that being empathetic also increases pro-social behavior in students, including helping others (Williams, O'Driscoll, and Moore 2014). Given that hate crimes still occur and that bullying is a major issue in many schools today, increasing empathy in students can help combat these societal problems.

When you think of empathy, you likely think of empathic concern, which entails social awareness in terms of being able to recognize another's emotional state, being in tune with the emotions of others, and feeling and showing concern if the emotions are negative or distressful. Empathic concern can also be taught, discussed, and developed in the classroom through a variety of activities.

Perspective Taking

Perspective taking is a cognitive form of empathy that relates to being able to take someone else's point of view. The idea is to put oneself in the shoes of another. In Harper Lee's *To Kill a Mockingbird*, Atticus Finch famously said, "You can never understand someone unless you understand their point of view, climb in that person's skin, or stand and walk in that person's shoes." While this is not typically what we think of when we think of empathy, it helps us better understand where someone is coming from. When we are able to understand others' perspectives, we are more likely to predict and evaluate others' emotions and responses and respect other people and the decisions they make.

Perspective taking is an excellent exercise to practice in the classroom. There are multiple opportunities to have students consider the perspectives of others; the following strategies can be incorporated through the content you are presenting to students.

Looking through Their Eyes

Have students consider the perspectives of different characters in a story or novel or discuss the perspective of a person in history. The following questions can help guide students:

- Why did _____ (the character or person) _____?
- What beliefs or values led them to _____?
- What events led to the character/person (taking an action) _____?
- What would you have done in that position?
- How do your values and beliefs differ from those of the character/person?
- What experiences have you had that are the same/similar/different?

By discussing a character's perspective, we open the door to having students consider the perspectives and motivations of others whom they encounter throughout their lives, including people they agree with and people they do not agree with.

Opposing Opinions

Current instructional standards focus on developing opinion and argumentative writing skills. Students are expected to clearly state their opinions and give reasons for them or state claims and provide evidence. As students build their own opinions and articulate reasons, they can share those opinions with others and learn about differing opinions. Similarly, as students begin to develop claims and provide evidence, they can learn to acknowledge counterclaims. Having students share these varied opinions and stances with others allows them to see diverse perspectives and prepares them to think about, analyze, and discuss important and sometimes controversial topics throughout their lives.

Tip!

Use children's literature to demonstrate perspective taking. Here are some suggestions:

I Will Fight Monsters for You by Santi Balmes, illustrated by Lyona: A young girl and a young monster have trouble sleeping because they are both afraid of each other.

Weird! (Book 1), *Dare!* (Book 2), and *Tough!* (Book 3) by Erin Frankel: Each book tells the story of bullying from three different perspectives: the target of bullying, the bystander, and the bully.

The Cat Who Lived with Anne Frank by David Lee Miller and Steven Jay Rubin: This book introduces the story of Anne Frank through the perspective of a cat.

💡 Fold the Line

A fun way for students to share their opinions or claims for an argument is to have them line up based on their viewpoints. Students line up and form a continuum from strongly agree to strongly disagree, with the people who feel the strongest one way or another on each end of the line. For example, with an opinion statement such as "Winter is the best season of the year," students would line up from strongly agree to strongly disagree, with varying levels of agreement in between.

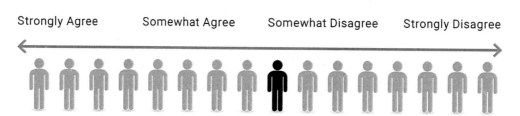

Once students are lined up, have them "fold the line" to meet with partners. Have the student in the middle of the line step forward and walk to one side of the line so that they are facing another student. The other students should follow the leader so that each student now has a partner.

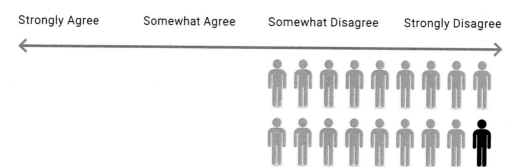

Note in this scenario that we have not folded the line from end to end, as that would have resulted in people with completely opposing positions standing face-to-face and people who are in the middle facing one another. By dividing the line in the center, we have people together whose viewpoints are not so far apart. Students can then discuss the differences in their opinions and learn the thoughts and perspectives of someone else.

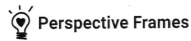

Perspective Frames

Using sentence frames or starters can be a helpful tool for students to discuss differing perspectives. By giving students some of the language needed, they can focus their attention on the various perspectives you would like them to consider. The following sentence frames are examples to help students discuss differing perspectives from a text, a video, or another student:

- The author wants me to learn (about) _____ (specific to nonfiction).
- I wonder why the author _____.
- I predict that the author's purpose is to inform/entertain/persuade because _____.
- After reading the selection, the author's purpose is _____ because _____.
- I think the author's purpose is _____ because _____.
- I am curious why the author _____.
- The main character _____. They did this by _____. They _____ did/did not do _____ because _____.
- _____ caused _____ because _____ happened.
- If _____, then _____.
- _____ occurred because _____.
- The effect of _____ was _____.
- The cause of _____ was _____.
- The character I most identify with is _____.
- The character I least identify with is _____.
- I can relate to this author because _____.
- If I had been _____, I would have _____ because _____.
- I think they might have felt _____.
- There are several clues that show us how they might have felt. One is _____.
- One way to interpret this event is _____.
- From their perspective, I think they were thinking _____.
- I already know that this person _____. To me, that means that they probably thought _____.

Divided Image

To use the Divided Image strategy, begin by finding a picture that is interesting and relates to the content students are studying. Print a large copy of the picture (or display it digitally) so that you can cut it into sections and still see the detail. Depending on the grade level and your desired outcome, the strategy can be completed in a variety of different ways.

Option 1: Cut the picture into sections. Each piece should show some detail from the picture. Distribute one section of the picture to each student. Have each student examine their section of the picture and draw or sketch to "complete" the picture with their predictions of what the rest of the picture would look like. Once completed, have students share their pictures in pairs or in small groups. Then reveal the original picture and have students find the section they had drawn and analyzed. Make sure to point out that each person had a piece of the picture, like a puzzle piece, and that what they looked at and drew or sketched represented their perspectives.

Option 2: Print the picture as large as possible and cut it into fourths; you should have one complete picture per group of four students. Place students into groups of four. Give one section of the picture to each student in the group. Have students discuss their section—what they see or observe in the picture and what they think the section represents or what the whole picture might be. Have students take turns sharing what they see without revealing their section. After each person has had a turn, have them each reveal their section, one at a time, and put the picture together as if it were a puzzle.

Option 3: Digitally project the image for the whole class, showing one section at a time. Have students discuss what they see in small groups or as a class. After each section is revealed, have students guess what is happening in the rest of the picture. Show the next section, and have them discuss it until you have shown each section. Then show the entire image.

Here is a sample image shown in four sections and the picture as a whole (see the next page). What would each student see, given the perspective they are shown? What assumptions might they make? When students see the picture as a whole and learn the history of the picture, how might their perspectives change?

Image 1

Image 2

Image 3

Image 4

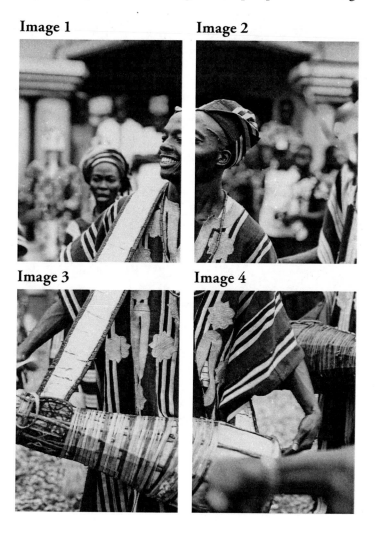

Complete Image

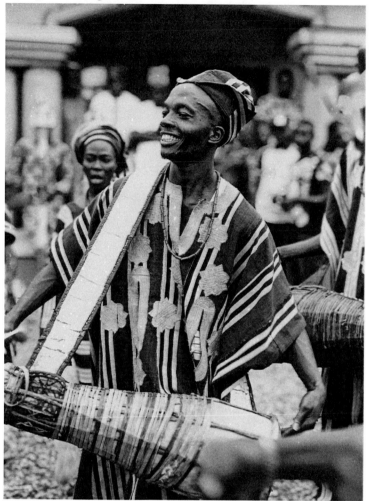

Yoruba bata drum players in Nigeria

After the exercise, have students discuss how their perspectives of the picture changed as they saw different sections. Did they automatically know what was happening in the picture after seeing the first section? If you use a historical picture or a picture representing a cultural practice that differs from that of the students, it can add a level of complexity to the discussion, as it may surprise students that what they perceived is quite different from what is actually happening in the picture.

Stop and Reflect

1. How does social awareness, or a lack thereof, manifest in your classroom? Think of a situation in which students did not have strong social-awareness skills and how it affected other students. Then reflect on a situation in which strong social-awareness skills played a role in a classroom scenario. What were the positive and negative aspects of those situations and scenarios?

2. Consider how social awareness can change the dynamic in your classroom, school, and community. Which strategies will you use to help students build deeper understandings of other people and their identities and cultures?

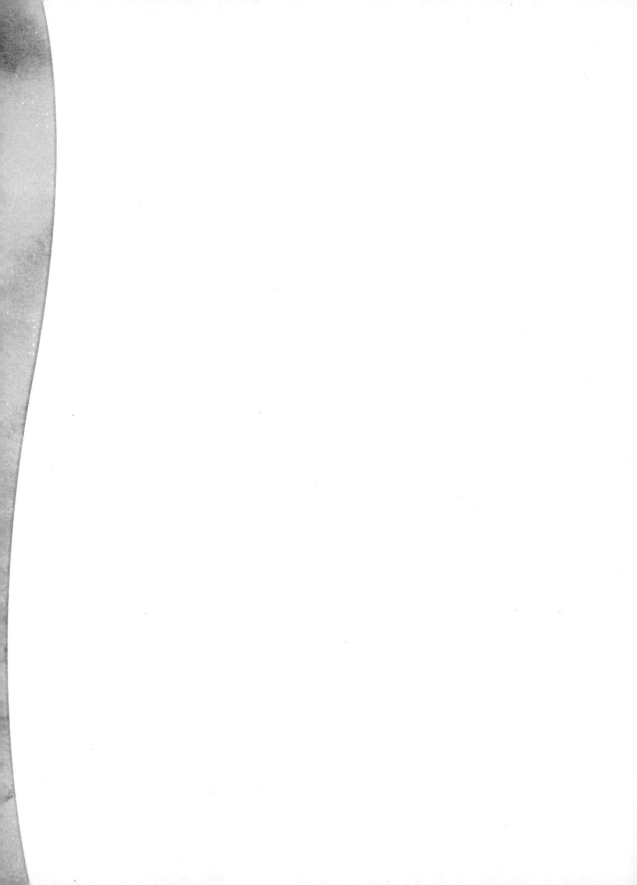

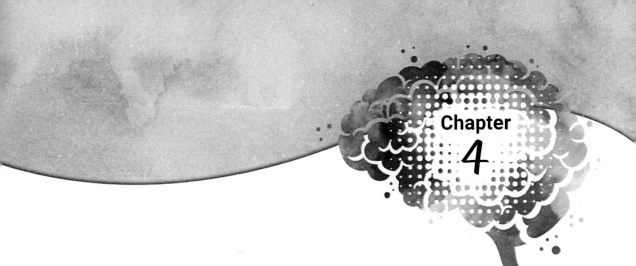

Relationship Skills

Defining Relationship Skills

Teaching and learning are social endeavors. In every classroom across the world, students and teachers get together to learn new information and skills. They do this through transmission of knowledge from the teacher to the student; through reading about events, stories, and other texts; by talking with one another and listening to differing perspectives; and by sharing their ideas through writing. At the heart of these activities are the relationships we build with one another. Students develop caring relationships with their teachers and teachers with their students. They respect one another and help one another grow. Students build respectful friendships with their peers, some of which will last a lifetime.

Relationships are a critical part of students' lives. While some of these relationships are of great importance, such as those with family members, others will be temporary. The word *relationship* is derived from the Latin word *relatus*, meaning "person related by blood or marriage" and from the Middle English suffix *–scheipe*, meaning "state or condition of being." Today, *relationship* can be defined as the way two or more people feel about and behave toward one another. Students need to learn how to manage the relationships they develop throughout their lives to have healthy and successful relationships.

People naturally develop relationships with others who are like them. It is normal for students to build relationships with the people who have one or more commonalities in terms of their identities, as they likely have similar values, beliefs, and behaviors. People with similar experiences naturally gravitate toward one another and build relationships.

Our biases, though, may also affect how we develop positive relationships with others. We may feel nervous or skeptical about people who are different from us, based on information (or misinformation) we have gotten through the media and society. When we begin to recognize that biases may affect how we view and treat others, we can begin to combat our biased thoughts and actions. These thoughts and actions may be subtle, so it is important to consistently monitor our thinking as we approach relationship development and management.

Learning about and getting to know people who are different from us is one of the richest experiences we can have, and it is a critical part of learning and development in school. As we learn about, build, and foster relationships, we also learn about the diversity of our world. As we develop positive relationships with others who are different from us, we also develop empathy and are less likely to engage in discriminatory, prejudiced, or biased behavior.

Of course, not all students develop friendships with one another. While learning is social, not all students get along. Conflicts in personalities, perspectives, and opinions can cause disruptions in the classroom and negatively affect the learning process. Some students have skills to resolve conflicts in appropriate and constructive ways, while others have not learned those skills.

Some students are more outgoing and extroverted, and some students are introverted and shy. Developing friendships and relationships will be easy for some and more challenging for others, for many reasons. Teachers can use a variety of strategies and activities to facilitate developing relationships and cultivate relationship management within the context of teaching content.

For some students, difficulty in building relationships may be related to a specific disability—for example, emotional disturbance. In the Individuals with Disabilities Education Act (IDEA), emotional disturbance is defined, in part, by an inability to build or maintain satisfactory interpersonal relationships with teachers or peers.

Teacher–Student Relationships

Teachers' relationships with students are important. It has been said that students may not remember everything we taught them, but they will remember how we made them feel. Teacher–student relationships affect just about every aspect of education, including students' well-being and academic achievement. As teachers, it is our responsibility to build and foster positive relationships with all students. They deserve to have a positive and healthy relationship with their teachers and know that they are respected for who they are.

There is significant research on the importance of teachers' relationships with students. When teachers have positive relationships with their students, students feel safe and supported in the learning environment, which ultimately leads to positive effects socially and academically (Baker, Grant, and Morlock 2008; O'Connor, Dearing, and Collins 2011; Silver et al. 2005).

Student–Student Relationships

All students already have a certain relationship when they enter the classroom—they are classmates. This is a superficial relationship level, but one that can be built on right at the start of the school year. Helping students use more specific vocabulary regarding their relationships can help them better manage those relationships and realize that relationships change over time. At times, we become closer to some people, and other times, we drift apart. Sometimes, our desire to be closer to someone is reciprocated, and sometimes it is not. Part of managing relationships is to be aware of this delicate balance and respond accordingly.

While it may not seem to be the explicit responsibility of a teacher to help students make friends, it is critical to help students establish respectful working relationships in the classroom and create a culture of learning. Students must be aware of their actions and feelings and emotions. They must learn to manage those actions, their facial expressions, and their postures and gestures (think back to the chapters on self-awareness and self-management), as these can have significant effects, both positive and negative, on relationships. Given that all students in your class have the relationship of being classmates, helping students establish deeper and better functioning relationships will help the classroom community be a place where students can focus more on learning and less on drama and conflict.

Modeling Positive Relationship Skills

The first step in teaching relationship skills to students is demonstrating how we use relationship skills in our everyday lives. This includes our relationships with colleagues, students' parents, and community members. Students should clearly see that we make efforts to get to know others and build relationships through strategies and tools, some of which are internalized and come naturally and others that are more conscious and intentional.

Teacher Authenticity

Having positive relationships with students does not mean we cannot have feelings. We are likely to get frustrated at times and be cheerful and content at other times. When we share our feelings with students, we demonstrate that we are human and that we have struggles and frustrations like everyone else. When we communicate these feelings, we show them that they are worthy of hearing about us, our thoughts, and our feelings.

Authenticity models what we want to see in students. Most of us do not like when we have ungenuine encounters with people—when someone acts one way but feels another way. This affects our interactions and may cause conflicts. While it takes a level of vulnerability to be authentic with students, it also shares your humanity and gives them permission to share theirs.

Listening to Students

"That teacher doesn't like me." Inevitably, teachers and administrators hear this from some students. Sometimes what students are referring to is feeling a lack of attention when they share something with a teacher. When students share information, even at incorrect times, we should be conscientious to acknowledge them and the information they shared. This can be done in a number of ways, including with looks or nods or, more overtly, by stating you heard them. You might answer the question immediately, ask that the student remind you about what they were sharing, or jot a note so that you can address it later.

Apologizing to Students

When we missed what a student said or perhaps said something we shouldn't have, we should apologize for it. Students should see that teachers can make mistakes, and when we do, we take responsibility for our mistakes and try to make it right—starting with an apology. It is critical that we apologize when we are wrong and to do so with sincerity.

One issue is that students may take offense to what we say or do based on their values, beliefs, and identities, which may be different from ours. We do not get to choose what offends others. We can, however, choose to take action when someone takes offense to something we have said or done. As language is constantly changing based on evolving understandings of people and identities, we may inadvertently say something that is considered offensive. At issue isn't political correctness but rather fostering relationships by apologizing as needed and changing as we learn more about students and communities.

Systems for Building Relationships

Another way to build, develop, and maintain relationships with students is to have a system of check-ins. Relationships are built and strengthened by consistent, caring contact. Regular check-ins show students that we care about them. You can use one or more variations, depending on the grade level, students' needs, and your schedule. Some check-ins are simple, such as greeting each student every day, and others are more complex. For example, you might greet students daily but use one-on-one check-ins to discuss issues that arise or need a more in-depth conversation.

Daily Greeting

Greeting students each day has multiple benefits, including developing and maintaining relationships with students. When we greet students, we are making a gesture to show them that they are important and that they matter. Research also shows that greeting students daily benefits their academic engagement by up to 20 percentage points and shows a 9 percent decrease in disruptive behavior (Cook et al. 2018). This leads to a net effect of an extra hour of learning time as a result of greeting students at the door each day.

The practice of greeting students can be integrated in several ways. Teachers can have students choose a handshake, high five, fist bump, hug, or wave, for example. Another fun alternative is to have students develop their own greetings and handshakes that they will perform with you at the door. It is important to include a variety of options to be culturally responsive and allow students to decide what feels best for them. A non-touch greeting can be included as an option, as some students may have sensory issues, may not want to be touched, or may prefer to wave on a given day.

As an alternative, you can have a designated student be the greeter for the day. Teach students the importance of greeting one another as a sign of respect, even if the other student is not a close friend.

In all cases, students should be greeted by their preferred names. Some students' legal or given names may differ from the names they use on a daily basis with family and friends. Ask students what name they prefer to be called, and use that name as a sign of respect and dignity. Some students' names may have originated from languages we do not speak and may be difficult to pronounce. It is vitally important that we learn to correctly pronounce students' names, and under no circumstances should we change or adapt students' names because we have difficulty pronouncing them. While we may never reach native-like fluency saying a student's name, we can ask the student, "Did I say your name correctly?" or "Teach me how to pronounce your name again, please," as a sign that we respect their identity.

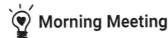 **Morning Meeting**

Class meetings can be effective ways to start or end your days. Celebrations, recognitions of accomplishments, problem-solving, or opportunities for reflection and sharing can be part of class meetings. For example, students can share good things that happened that day or the previous day. Students can take turns sharing by passing an object or being called on one by one to share important news, events, or ideas.

You can present a problem occurring in the classroom, the school, or the world, and students can brainstorm potential solutions to the problem. This provides students the opportunity to share ideas as well as hear from other students in the class.

Here are some other ideas to include in a morning meeting:

▸ **Peaks and Pits:** Students share peaks, or successes, accomplishments, or positive aspects of their lives, either academic or social. As students share their peaks, the other students can offer celebration statements. Students may also share their pits—challenges or hard things that have happened—and the other students can offer words of acknowledgment and encouragement. Often, by acknowledging that what a person is sharing is a challenge validates and affirms students. *Optional:* Have students do a quick-write or quick-draw of their peaks and pits in preparation to share at the morning meeting.

▸ **Great News! Guess What?** Students share good things that are happening in their lives or that have happened during the day. This can be anything they would like to share with others in the class.

▸ **Pass It!** Use a large beach ball with questions written on it, a number cube, or another object with numbers or questions written on it. One student starts by tossing the ball; the student who catches it answers the question that their right thumb (or other finger) touches. Alternatively, a student rolls the number cube and answers the corresponding question. Some sample questions include the following:

   ❏ What is something you love?

   ❏ What is something that bothers you?

   ❏ What is something you are happy about?

   ❏ Who helped you recently?

   ❏ What is a goal you are working on?

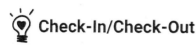 **Check-In/Check-Out**

The check-in/check-out system is designed to provide an opportunity to check in with someone at the beginning of the day or week and to check out with them at the end of the day or week. This system allows students to talk to someone in the morning, preferably before school starts. During the check-in, students can share how they are feeling, share any challenges for the day or week, set goals, or discuss anything on their minds. At the end of the day or week, students check-out with the same person. Students can share what happened, ways they self-managed, progress made toward goals, or any other topics.

It's important to keep in mind that not all students need the check-in/check-out system. While all students can benefit from establishing a relationship with someone in the school, it may be that your school does not have the resources to implement such a program. It should be noted that the person the student is checking in with does not have to be the student's teacher. In fact, it can be helpful for the student to establish a relationship with another adult in the building, including any of the following:

- Administrators
- Custodians
- Cafeteria workers
- Coaches
- Secretaries
- Older students who have been trained

The check-in/check-out system can be formalized with sign-in sheets—documents that students use to record information and that their partners will sign. A variety of topics can be included on the form, such as a scale of how students are feeling at the beginning or end of the day, challenges that arose, and successes and accomplishments. These forms serve as written records for students and parents over the course of the year. The following form is an example of what a check-in/check-out form can look like, adapted from the work of Jim Wright (n.d.) at Intervention Central. For additional examples, see the Digital Resources.

> **Competency Connections**
> The check-in/check-out system also deepens self-awareness and helps students to self-manage as they plan for and reflect on their own behaviors, specific goals, or ways they are coping with challenges in their lives.

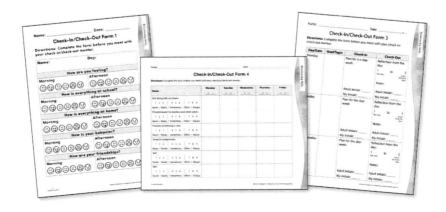

Sample Check-In/Check-Out Form

Day/Date	Goal/Topic	Check-In	Check-Out
Monday	Getting along with others	Plan for the day/week: Adult Initials: _____ Student Initials: _____	Reflection from the day: 1 to 5 Not met most/all of the time Notes: Adult Initials: _____ Student Initials: _____
Tuesday	Showing kindness to someone	Plan for the day/week: Adult Initials: _____ Student Initials: _____	Reflection from the day: 1 to 5 Not met most/all of the time Notes: Adult Initials: _____ Student Initials: _____
Wednesday	Reflecting on gratitude	Plan for the day/week: Adult Initials: _____ Student Initials: _____	Reflection from the day: 1 to 5 Not met most/all of the time Notes: Adult Initials: _____ Student Initials: _____

Continued

Sample Check-In/Check-Out Form *(cont.)*

Day/Date	Goal/Topic	Check-In	Check-Out
Thursday	Apologizing to someone	Plan for the day/week: Adult Initials: _____ Student Initials: _____	Reflection from the day: 1 to 5 Not met most/all of the time Notes: Adult Initials: _____ Student Initials: _____
Friday	Letting go of things that are bothering me	Plan for the day/week: Adult Initials: _____ Student Initials: _____	Reflection from the day: 1 to 5 Not met most/all of the time Notes: Adult Initials: _____ Student Initials: _____

Alternative Meeting Times

Sometimes, teachers are able to allow students into their classroom before school starts or have "office hours" where they can work informally with students. These extra meeting times, where students are able to interact with the teacher and with one another, provide excellent opportunities to informally build relationships. While it is not always possible or practical to have students come into your classroom during these times or to meet with students individually, any opportunity we can find to meet with students can help deepen relationships.

At the middle and high school levels, this extra meeting time can take the form of an advisory period. The advisory period or homeroom can be used for a variety of topics, and an excellent use of time is including activities that help build, foster, and deepen relationships with students.

Team-Building Activities

Team-building activities can be used any time to help establish a culture and community of trust and learning to help students build and maintain relationships. There are many types of team-building activities, including icebreakers and warm-ups, name games, collaboration activities, communication practice activities, problem-solving games, and more.

These activities can get students ready for the day or for the class period, as brain breaks, or at the end of class. The activities can be linked to content so that students are not only getting to know one another and building positive relationships but also practicing content knowledge in a different way.

Icebreakers and Warm-Ups

Icebreakers are designed to help students get to know one another or get them ready to work together. Icebreakers can be used at various times, including at the start of the school year, when a new group of students gathers together, or throughout the year to continue to deepen relationships. Effective icebreakers allow students to meet and greet one another and learn new things about their partners. Here are a variety of icebreaker and team-building activities that can be used with groups of any size (adapted from Teampedia.net).

- **Cup O' Questions:** Brainstorm simple questions or provide a list of questions that students can answer quickly. Write the questions on slips of paper and put them in a box or container. This is the Cup O' Questions. Choose a student and have them pull a question out of the Cup O' Questions. The student must answer that question. When they are done, either add the question back into the container or remove that question. The following are some suggested questions. Additional questions can be found in the Digital Resources.

  ❏ What is your favorite food?

  ❏ What is a food you will NOT eat?

  ❏ If you could be any animal, which would it be, and why?

  ❏ What is one thing you love to do?

  ❏ What is your favorite place?

Tip!

Provide students with a time frame to answer the question. If you are unable to get to every student on the same day, record which students have shared so that everyone gets a turn to answer one of the questions in the Cup O' Questions.

- **Going on a Picnic!** Have students stand in a circle as a whole class or in smaller groups. Have the first person state their name along with the name of a food they would bring on a picnic. The name of the food must begin with first letter of the person's name. For example, "I'm Erick, and I'm bringing eggplant." The following students have to state the names and foods of the people who went before them before sharing their names. "Erick is bringing eggplant. I'm Sandra, and I am bringing salad." For an added challenge, change the topic to something content related and have students brainstorm vocabulary that starts with the first letter of their first or last names.

- **Creative Handshakes:** Place students in pairs. Have each pair develop a creative handshake that they will use to great each other. The handshakes can be as simple or as elaborate as desired. Encourage students to have two, three, or more moves to the handshake. Once pairs have memorized their handshakes, have them split up and meet with someone new. The new pairs then take turns teaching their handshakes to their new partners.

Task Teams

Task Teams are a way to bring students together in the classroom to promote collaboration, communication, and relationship-building skills. They typically comprise a heterogeneous group of four students—one who is high achieving, two who are average achieving, and one who is lower achieving—who sit near one another. Task Teams work together on a variety of tasks, including reading to one another, completing group projects, or working with cooperative learning structures. The idea is that each student benefits from having the other students in the group. Outside of Task Teams, the teacher can pull homogeneous groups of students for other purposes.

To support relationship building, Task Teams should develop team names. While students may want to choose silly names or names based purely on popular culture, an activity that helps strengthen relationships is to have students brainstorm common characteristics. To do this, students create a chart with three or more columns. The first column includes characteristics that are unique to one individual in the group. The second column identifies characteristics shared by two people, the third column identifies characteristics shared by three people, and so on. Once students have generated a list together, they will develop team names based on the commonalities shared by the group.

Students can brainstorm any number of characteristics. Some simple characteristics include the following:

- Number of siblings
- Birth month
- Likes/dislikes: foods, movies, music, book genres, games, or sports

Three-Step Interview

The Three-Step Interview is an activity that encourages students to get to know partners as they practice an interview format. Students can also use the interviews with content-area learning to quiz one another on content, share their opinions, make predictions, or share background knowledge and experiences around the topic being studied. This strategy is most interesting when students are paired with others they don't know as well.

Step One: Students are paired up; one student will start as the interviewer and one as the interviewee. Students discuss the questions posed in an interview format.

Step Two: Switch roles. After a set amount of time, the person who was being interviewed now becomes the interviewer.

Step Three: Form small groups of four and share. Have two pairs of students team up to introduce their partners and share the information they learned from the person they interviewed.

 ## Find Someone Who

The Find Someone Who activity provides a way for students to interact with someone else in the classroom based on specific criteria. Any number of criteria can be used. The following are examples that can be used with any grade level; you can adapt them to fit students' needs:

Find someone who _____.

> - is wearing the same color as you
> - has the same number of siblings as you
> - was born in the same month as you
> - enjoys an activity you do (reading, writing, the same genre of movie, playing a particular sport or game, etc.)

Follow these steps for the Find Someone

Add Greetings

To add a fun and interesting element to the Find Someone Who activity, students can engage in a particular greeting when they meet with someone. Students can practice both formal and informal greetings, depending on the situation. For example, have students engage in formal greetings by having them shake hands when they find their partners. Then have them exchange verbal greetings, such as "Hello. How do you do?" For informal greetings, students can give high-fives or fist bumps and add verbal exchanges such as "What's up?"

Who activity:

1. Create a discussion question or activity that students will engage in.

2. Share the question or activity directions with students.

3. Decide how many students will be in a group: two, three, or four.

4. Explain that they will be looking for other students who meet the criterion you call out. The only caveat is they can't meet with their nearest classmates.

5. Have students stand up and push in their chairs. Share that at your signal, they will need to find someone who _____. Provide students with the criterion for meeting with someone else in the room.

6. Provide a specific time frame for students to find partners (or small groups).

7. Give students the signal to go find partners or small groups who match the criterion you provided. Once students have found their partners, they will start working on the assigned activity or discussion.

Collaborative Learning to Build Relationships

Collaborative learning involves students working together to practice the information being taught. Although some believe that collaborative learning means putting students into groups and having them work together, this is only a small part of collaborative learning; group work and collaborative learning are not the same. In traditional group work, there may not be explicit structures to ensure all students are involved and held accountable. In other words, if one person can do all or most of the work while others minimally participate, it is not collaborative learning!

Collaborative learning builds a number of skills, including the ability to work with others, resolve conflict, delegate tasks, and take responsibility. These are key elements of success in today's workplace, as students will work with diverse groups of people in their lifetimes. As students work together to accomplish a goal or complete a task, they are also learning about different ways of thinking and completing tasks, learning ways to manage time, and learning about the strengths of others.

Cooperative learning, as described by Spencer Kagan in *Cooperative Learning* (1994), involves the following key elements, outlined by the acronym PIES:

- ▶ Positive interdependence
- ▶ Individual accountability
- ▶ Equitable participation
- ▶ Simultaneous interaction

Each of these elements is designed to help students work in diverse teams, accomplish a group goal of completing an activity or task, and manage relationships with the other team members. Let's now look at each of those elements in more detail.

Positive Interdependence

Positive interdependence is critical to cooperative learning. Cooperative learning requires cooperation and positive interdependence. Students need one another to complete the task; one student cannot complete the task without the others. There are several ways to create positive interdependence among students working in cooperative groups.

Part to Whole

One way to create positive interdependence is to create tasks in which each student must contribute a unique part for the task to be completed. Each student in the group has a specific portion of the task to contribute or has information that the other team members do not have but that is needed to complete the task. This can be accomplished through task cards or through small-group instruction, wherein each member of a team receives different information from the teacher. Students are responsible for relaying that information back to their teams and working to put all the parts together to complete the task or assignment.

Student Roles

Another way to build positive interdependence among students is to give them specific roles within the group. This helps students stay engaged in the task, as they have something specific that they have to do. Students can play many roles in cooperative groups in the classroom, including the following:

- ▸ **Team Leader:** ensures that the team is working toward the goals and that each person is fulfilling their role in the group
- ▸ **Timer:** keeps the group focused on the time they have to complete the task and monitors the progress of the group in relation to the remaining time
- ▸ **Recorder:** takes notes and records information for the group as a whole (each student may still be responsible for individual note-taking or other writing opportunities)
- ▸ **Reporter/Presenter:** shares with the whole group/class at designated times, reporting the content discussed, progress made, and so on
- ▸ **Resource Monitor:** gets, distributes, and otherwise manages the materials needed for each activity
- ▸ **Errand Monitor:** runs errands for the group, including checking in with other groups for clarification, asking the teacher questions, and so on
- ▸ **Questioner/Skeptic:** asks questions to challenge the thinking of the group and/or to provide other perspectives
- ▸ **Encourager/Coach:** ensures that all are participating, encourages others to participate, compliments group members on their contributions, and so on
- ▸ **Reflector:** observes and notes the strengths and areas of growth in terms of group dynamics and progress on the project or activity
- ▸ **Harmonizer:** helps resolve conflicts among the group and ensures that each student is respectful to others
- ▸ **Innovator:** brings new ideas to the group that may have been heard or shared by other groups or helps implement ideas from other students in the group

Having specific roles and the opportunity to work on team tasks should be coupled with the next key element of cooperative learning: individual accountability.

Individual Accountability

While each student is responsible for adding some piece to the task, each student must be held responsible for their work, and the other members of the team should not be punished if one member did not finish. For example, if students are filling in a story map, completing a team graphic organizer, or writing a story or essay together, each student is required to add a specific section or piece to the assignment and will be held accountable for doing so.

Equitable Participation

Along with individual accountability, students should have roughly equal participation in the tasks. However, we can differentiate for students by having a variety of ways students can contribute to the task. Equitable participation means that all students have the opportunity to contribute to the task in ways that are challenging and allow them to stretch their learning. It does not mean that each student has to do the exact same thing or an exactly equal amount; each student should contribute in a way that makes sense for that particular student.

Simultaneous Interaction

Interaction is key in collaborative learning, just as it is in relationships. Students should have the opportunity to work with one another simultaneously so that they can process information, solve problems, and practice using academic language. As students are able to share space, they are also developing and deepening relationships with one another, working toward a common purpose. Simultaneous interaction is achieved when students work together in small groups. For example, if you have students in groups of four, and one student per group is talking, then one fourth of the class is talking and interacting with their team members.

Communication Skills to Build Relationships

Communication is an essential skill for all people. Our need to communicate thoughts, ideas, and needs is deeply rooted in the human experience. Communication, essentially, is the transmission of information, including feelings, thoughts, perceptions, expectations, commands, attitudes, knowledge, and more. Effective communication is at the cornerstone of relationship building and relationship management. Communication has a few basic requirements: an idea or message, a sender, and a receiver. Once the idea or message has been identified (this may be instantaneous or unconscious), the sender must encode the message. This involves conscious and unconscious processing in the brain. The sender then delivers the message, and the receiver must then decode the message or interpret the meaning. Most people have had an experience where a miscommunication led to frustrating or embarrassing results. It may have been at work, with a loved one, or with a friend. In any circumstance, it is favorable to have clear, concise communication.

Accepting *No* for an Answer

This can be difficult for people at any age. Yet there are many times in life when we must accept that we can't always get our way. For students, it may be that they want to play a game with a group, join a group of students for a project, or ask to borrow materials. It is important for students to understand they may hear *no* sometimes and that how they respond can affect the relationship they have with the other person.

Here are some ways students can practice accepting *no* for an answer:

▸ **Acknowledge the person** by saying "OK" and find an alternative. For younger students especially, the teacher may need to provide some alternatives. Alternative actions may include using other materials, engaging in a different activity, or using a self-management strategy to focus and calm down.

▸ **Play "May I Please...?** The goal of the game is to move from one area of the room to another. One person is at one end, and the group is at another. The leader may begin by saying, "Some of you may take three steps forward." Each group member then must ask, "May I please take three (large/small/baby/dancing/etc.) steps?" The leader has the choice of responding *yes* or *no* to each student. If students move forward without saying, "May I please...?" they must return to the starting line.

▸ **Collaboratively brainstorm** times that students have been told *no*, either by caregivers or friends. Then have them discuss how they reacted and what the best way to react would be in a particular situation.

Giving and Getting Feedback

Students need to learn to get and give effective feedback in the classroom. They will receive feedback from teachers based on behavior and academics. Students can give their peers feedback, too. When providing feedback, it is helpful for students to consider positive feedback first and to be as specific as possible. Model for students how to provide specific positive feedback on an assignment, for example.

- ▸ **Start positive:** Have students share what they liked or something that was powerful, effective, important, interesting, and so on.

- ▸ **Be specific:** Have students use phrases such as "I liked the part when you _____," "The details you added about _____ were clear and specific," or "_____ was very effective because _____." General feedback, such as "I liked it," is not very effective; by adding *because* to a statement, we build in specificity.

- ▸ **Use constructive language:** As students give feedback on what can be changed, suggestions should be stated clearly. For example, if a prompt or a rubric lists specific criteria, feedback should be based on the criteria. If the assignment is missing something, the person providing feedback should clearly state that with phrases such as "The rubric states we need three details, and I only see two. You need to add one more to meet the standards." Suggestions can be made using phrases such as "You might consider _____," "Have you tried _____?" or "Have you thought about _____?" The person receiving the feedback should then thank the person for their suggestions and the feedback they have given.

- ▸ **Use responsible choice:** It is important that students know that giving and getting feedback is meant to be helpful and designed to support them and their peers in improving their work. Collaborating and sharing our thoughts builds relationships. It is, however, the choice of the person receiving the feedback to change their work or to leave the work as it was created. Each person has the responsibility to choose what to do with the feedback they have been given.

Expressing Frustration

Everyone gets frustrated. When we do, it is important to express that frustration in a way that develops and maintains our relationships. One way students can learn to express frustration is by using *I* statements. To use an *I* statement, students can use the following formula:

I feel + (name of feeling/emotion) + because _____.

This sentence frame puts the feeling or emotion first, thereby focusing on the person and the effect rather than the particular action.

Expressing Disagreement

The key to maintaining relationships when there are disagreements is to be respectful. Nobody has to agree with everything all the time. However, when there is respect, people can peacefully disagree and express their disagreement in ways that value the other person and their points of view. Students can use the following phrases and sentence frames to respectfully disagree with others:

- ▶ I disagree because _____.
- ▶ I respectfully disagree because _____.
- ▶ That's not how I see it. I think _____.
- ▶ Another way to look at this is _____.
- ▶ Another perspective to consider is _____.
- ▶ I don't agree/I partially agree with your point about _____ because _____.
- ▶ I have a different way of looking at/thinking about this because _____.
- ▶ I agree in part with your idea, but I was also thinking _____.
- ▶ I understand what you're saying, but I think it means _____.
- ▶ I'd like to suggest a different idea: _____.

Respecting Diverse Viewpoints

We live in a diverse world. People will have varying viewpoints and interpretations based on their values, cultures, backgrounds, and experiences. It is important for students to realize that these viewpoints are not wrong but rather different from theirs. When viewpoints are significantly different and difficult to understand, students can use perspective-taking strategies such as pausing, suspended disbelief, or using questioning skills to better understand another person's viewpoints.

When we ask questions with authenticity and genuine curiosity, it shows the other person that we are interested in what they have to say. The question stems on the following page may help students share their perspectives with one another.

- What makes you think that?
- Why do you feel that way?
- What could I have done differently?
- What would you do in my situation?
- What ideas do you have?
- Tell me more about your idea.

Kindness and Gratitude: Key Relationship Skills

Kindness and gratitude are two keys to starting, developing, and fostering any strong relationship. These exercises can be implemented either formally or informally to encourage students to demonstrate kindness and express gratitude.

 Kindness Wall

With this strategy, students write examples of kindness that they have seen throughout the day on sticky notes and stick them to the Kindness Wall. This can be anonymous, or they can include names of people who demonstrated kindness.

 Kindness Bingo

To play Kindness Bingo, students brainstorm various ways they can demonstrate kindness over the course of a week. Bingo cards are created (either by you or students), and students engage in acts of kindness over a week. Students can choose the squares, or you can select a few activities that students must engage in to earn a mark on the bingo board. While a game such as bingo implies that students will get a prize, no specific prizes are necessary, as the demonstration of kindness and its benefits are the prizes! Sample Kindness Bingo cards can be found in the Digital Resources.

Appreciations and Shout-Outs

With this strategy, students have opportunities to show appreciation and gratitude on a daily or weekly basis. This can be done formally, such as during a certain time every day, or on an informal basis, such as when there are a few minutes during a transition or at the end of class. All you have to do is open the floor to anyone who would like to give an appreciation or a shout-out to a classmate, school staff member, or another student. Alternatively, you can designate a specific day of the week, such as Thankful Thursdays, to allow students to share their appreciations and shout-outs. Adding hand gestures, such as a round of applause, a thumbs up, or a fireworks clap, make the shout-outs even more fun.

Gratitude Journals

Journals are excellent tools to help students build writing skills and express and reflect on gratitude. This could include being grateful for people in their lives, things that have happened, or kindness others have shown them. Entries in the journal can be formatted in a variety of ways.

- ▶ **Three Good Things:** Students write three things or people they are grateful for.
- ▶ **Letter of Thanks:** Students write formatted letters expressing gratitude. These letters can be sent or kept private and can be written to anyone, including themselves, people they know, historical people, or fictional characters.

- **Helping Hands:** Students record ways in which people have helped them or been kind to them recently. In addition, they can add how they have been helpful to others and how that made them feel, or how they might be helpful to other people in the coming days.

- **Lessons Learned:** Students share ideas about things that they learned to do that were challenging or difficult but that they are grateful to have learned.

- **That's Funny!** Students reflect on things that made them laugh recently. This might include jokes, books or movies, or situations that made them chuckle.

- **Looking Ahead:** Students share exciting or fun events they are looking forward to.

- **I've Got Personality:** Students share aspects of their character or personality traits that they are grateful for or have helped them.

Relationship Management through Conflict Resolution

A conflict occurs when there is a disagreement or problem among two or more people. Every person will experience conflict in their life as they work with and get to know other people. It is not inherently wrong or problematic to have conflict. The question is how do we deal with the conflicts we encounter? Conflict often starts small but can grow more problematic if not dealt with appropriately. For students, learning how to peacefully and effectively resolve conflicts helps them build relationship skills and effectively manage their relationships.

Small groups are a powerful place to practice conflict resolution skills. The following plan can be used as is or modified to fit students' needs.

- Bring the involved students together in a neutral place. Consider using a conference room or another teacher's classroom.

- Begin by asking students if they agree to solve the problem. If all parties agree, explain the process to students. You might consider having them sign an agreement that states they are willing to solve the problem at hand.

- Explain that each person will have an opportunity to share their perspective. During this time, the other student(s) will only listen and not respond in the moment.

- After each person has shared, potential solutions will be discussed. Solutions can be suggested by the person facilitating the meeting (an adult or another student trained in the process) or by the participating students.

- Together, students should agree on one or more of the solutions. Students can sign an agreement form stating that they agree to implement the solution.

Conflict is an inevitable part of being human. Students should understand and learn that they can deal with conflict in healthy ways that strengthen their relationships with others. Conflict is meant to be worked through. Sometimes the process is challenging and takes time. But as we learn to address conflict, we are better able to build and maintain our relationships with others and solve problems together.

> **Competency Connections**
>
> Conflict resolution is also an aspect of responsible decision-making. When students solve conflicts that have arisen—even small ones—they are prepared to tackle challenges that have larger implications for their lives and for society. Allowing conflicts to fester not only disrupts relationships but also can have a negative effect on our health, the health of others, and on society.

Tips for Maintaining Relationships

We take many actions to foster and maintain positive relationships every day. These can be pointed out to students and practiced in the classroom.

Be Supportive: In any type of relationship, it is important to support each other. This may be through helping someone when they need it or by being there to listen. Here are some statements and questions students can use to show support:

- I'm here for you.
- How can I help you?
- What do you need right now?
- How can I support you?
- I am here to listen anytime.

Be Encouraging: We can provide encouragement to each other in times of success and hardship. Here are some statements that help provide encouragement:

- I'm proud of you.
- That was fantastic!
- It was great how you _____.
- You made great strides!
- You're getting better each time you try!

Do Not Tease or Belittle: At times, friends poke fun at each other. However, it can be easy for students to unknowingly cross a line and make a person feel bad. When students have social awareness, they will notice when their playfulness is turning into something harmful. Here are some statements that students can use when they feel belittled or teased:

- Please stop.
- That's enough.
- I don't appreciate that.
- You are going too far.
- You are making me feel bad. It was funny at first, but it's not anymore.

Compromise: Compromise can be a challenging skill for students. Depending on students' ages, they may not have learned sharing and compromising skills. Here are some simple ideas to help students compromise:

- How about if this time we _____ , and next time we can _____.
- How might we combine these ideas into one?
- Can you live with doing it this way?

Be Considerate: Everyone appreciates it when someone is considerate of their needs, likes, and opinions. We can be considerate of others by first observing others we care about. When we are observant, we notice things about the person, such as their likes and dislikes. We can continue by making a conscious effort to think about and acknowledge others. From there, we can make gestures or verbalize that we are thinking of the other person. Here are some phrases that may show consideration:

- I noticed that you seem to like/dislike _____.
- I thought of you when _____.
- I thought you might like _____.

Stop and Reflect

1. Consider students you have strong, healthy relationships with. What contributed to developing and fostering those relationships?

2. Now, consider a student or students you do not have that same level of relationship with. What strategies can you use to develop deeper relationships with those students?

3. Think about your classroom and your class (or classes). What is the overall climate? Do all students have healthy and respectful relationships with one another? What relationship skills need to be continued, fostered, and developed? Which strategies will you incorporate to teach students relationship skills?

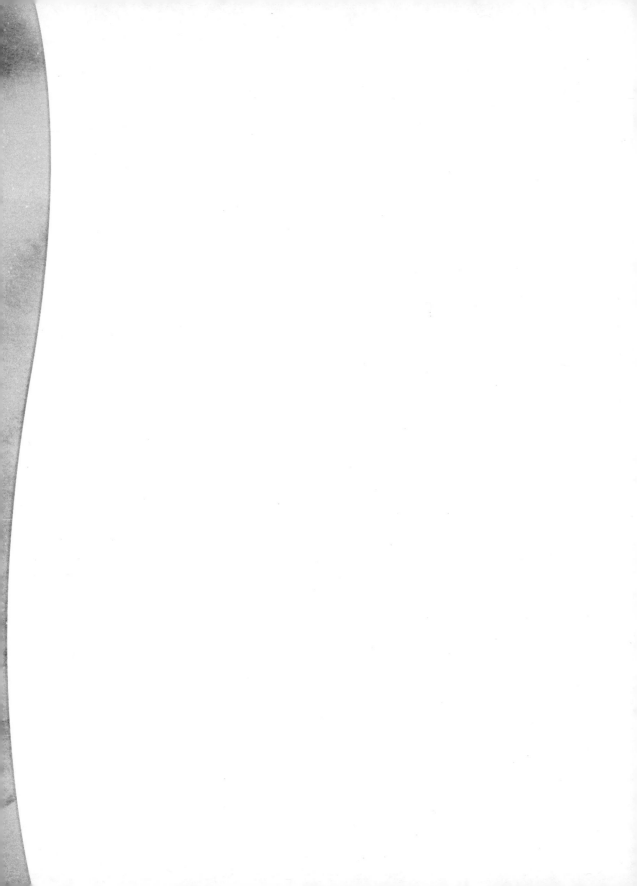

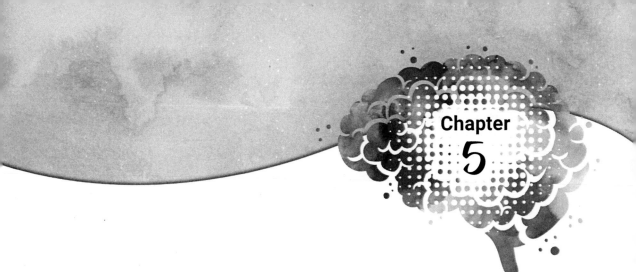

Responsible Decision-Making

Defining Responsible Decision-Making

Each day, we make thousands of choices; some of them are subconscious, and others we are keenly aware of. Many of our choices lead to positive outcomes, but some do not! To make decisions, people need to consider a variety of factors, including their own values and concerns, the various choices available, and what the consequences of those choices might be.

As teachers, we make many professional decisions on a daily basis: decisions about what and how to teach, what to say or not to say to students and colleagues, how to manage our classrooms, and more. We also are aware of student choices and how those affect us and the other students in the classroom. Responsible decision-making on the part of students helps keep the classroom running smoothly and helps with classroom management. We are all aware, however, that some students have difficulty making responsible decisions. We may see that students are impulsive, decide not to make good choices, or follow what others do without thought.

Given all this, we can certainly take actions to help students make responsible decisions in the classroom. Students should first understand that making decisions for themselves is a fundamental human right and that they can and will need to take responsibility for the decisions they make. They also need to realize that good outcomes are not guaranteed by good decisions, but a good decision will make sense to them and feel right. As teachers, we can also provide opportunities to pause before deciding or acting, to think it through and then decide. While we cannot control what students do outside the classroom, equipping them with the skills to make responsible decisions will serve them throughout their lives.

The Decision for Social Justice

Social justice is one of the key aspects of education—making the world a better place for every individual and every group of people. Given the continued events and acts of violence, bigotry, racism, and hatred, we must teach students that these topics are not just things we observe or discuss; we must make the decision to act as responsible citizens of the world to combat injustice and hatred.

To do this, we can begin with discussions of current and past world events, including incidents from our own lives, communities, and classrooms. Depending on students' ages, it may not be appropriate to discuss issues of violence. However, we can discuss issues of fairness, justice, and bias that are happening around us. Many children's books depict events and attitudes that have affected people negatively. Bringing student awareness to these issues and discussing the actions they can take, or the actions others could have taken, will help bring the issues to light.

As we discuss these issues more regularly with students, we will have the opportunity to share strategies for combating injustice. For example, students may ask about what to do when they hear comments that are offensive, especially when they are racist or bigoted in nature. One strategy is to "call out" people for making such comments and let them know that those comments are unwelcome and unacceptable. While this is important, it may be even more critical that we "call in" people,

Competency Connections

When students are self-aware, they can more clearly articulate their identities, values, and beliefs. As they develop deeper social awareness, they learn about different perspectives from others. When people have values and beliefs that differ significantly or are offensive, self-management helps us respond in ways that allow us to grow and learn. We can then build relationships with people who are different from us and learn from them. As these pieces come together, we make responsible decisions that benefit everyone.

or help them understand why their comments are hurtful, unwelcomed, and unacceptable. In this way, we do not just condemn people but educate them. At the same time, we don't allow comments that disparage the identity of others.

We also must teach students to act in the face of hate. We can help students understand that they can fight issues such as prejudice and hate in many ways. While it may not be safe to directly address a person or group in a rage, students can act when they see microaggressions and hold themselves and others accountable when they encounter situations that negatively affect others. Students can act in these ways:

▶ Directly addressing comments that disparage others and their identities

▶ Reporting acts that harm others to someone in authority

▶ Not engaging in behaviors that negatively affect others

The first step is to not shy away from the topic of responsibility to combat violence, bigotry, racism, and injustice. We must make conscious decisions to work toward a world in which injustice, hatred, bigotry, and racism are eliminated.

Teaching Responsible Decision-Making

Teaching responsible decision-making involves multiple steps. Some steps will depend on students' ages and grade levels. Perhaps the first and simplest step we can take is to create classroom guidelines that encourage responsible decisions. Our classroom rules and procedures may include some level of choice. In addition, you can remind students throughout the day to make responsible decisions. For example, when you are getting ready to do an activity, remind students that a responsible decision is to wait to start after they hear all directions. Some students will be tempted to get materials out as you are talking and not pay attention to all the directions. If students are to move somewhere in the classroom, such as to get additional materials, come to a carpet area, or meet in groups, they may begin to move before you have given complete directions. Students may need to be reminded that they should stand up, push in their chairs, and walk calmly through the classroom. These simple reminders and the phrase "Make a responsible decision by _____" serve as a guide about appropriate decisions.

You can certainly remind students that a particular decision they are making is not helpful, appropriate, or responsible. In this case, you might say, "What you are doing right now is not a responsible decision (or a good choice). Please make a responsible decision and _____." It is important that you provide an alternative for the student. Just telling the student to make a responsible decision may not be helpful, as they may not know what a responsible decision would be. Consider the following classroom scenarios and how the teacher provided the opportunity for students to make responsible decisions.

Scenario for Young Students

A student is so fidgety that they cannot seem to sit still. As you are giving directions, the student is bouncing in their chair, waving their hands about, tapping the desk, and distracting others. Your first impulse is to say in a stern voice, "Please stop! Sit still. You are distracting others, and they will not know what to do because you are getting them off track!" But you realize from experience that this is not the best decision, as it will only draw more attention to the student and distract the rest of the class. Moreover, when you have done that in the past, it worked only for a few seconds, and shortly after your comments were made, the student began to bounce around and distract people again.

You decide to walk over to the student to use proximity as a tool to help the student focus. You put your hand on their shoulder to calm them for a moment. Later that day, you talk with the student about their behavior and how it was distracting others. Together, you brainstorm some tools the student can use to self-manage when they are feeling energetic during quiet time. You decide together that when you notice that the student is especially energetic, you will provide them with a squishy ball to squeeze under the table to relieve some energy. You also decide to install a rubber band between the legs of the chair, using an old bicycle tire, so that the student can press on the band with their feet without distracting others. You then discuss that you will try these tools for two weeks to see if they help the student make better decisions and self-manage during instructional time.

Scenario for Older Students

A pair of students are disrupting the class, whispering to each other during instructional time. You say, "Excuse me! You are being very rude by talking while I am talking. Make a good decision and stay quiet so that you can pay attention." The students rebut that they were just trying to get clarification from a classmate on something that was confusing. You then begin to tell them that the timing was inappropriate and that they should wait until you finish to raise their hands and ask for clarification. Again, the students have a response to argue with you, complaining that you are unclear and that they need help.

You then realize that telling them to make a responsible decision was confusing, as they were indeed making a responsible decision by trying to get clarification. The issue is that they were talking out of turn and potentially disturbing the class. Instead, provide two options that students can use to signal you when they are confused and need clarification. One option is to use a set of three cards—green, yellow, and red—that each student will have on their desks. Students can use these cards at any time to indicate their levels of understanding. Students can also use sticky notes to jot questions or write a question mark and stick them on the edge of the desk. As you scan the room, when you see a sticky note on the side of a desk, you can pause and have students check in with each other through a short peer-to-peer discussion, and you can check in with students individually.

The Decision-Making Process

For many students, making decisions seems like an abstract concept with no real process attached to it. It is important to help students learn that there is an actual process they can follow to help them evaluate choices and make responsible decisions.

You can begin by modeling the decision-making process authentically by walking students through the process you take when making decisions in the classroom. These decisions can range from instructional decisions to intentional scheduling changes to decisions to seize on a teachable moment. Share with students your thought process as you make the decision, and be as explicit as possible about the process. This can be as simple as telling students the considerations you took as you made a decision.

As you continue to "pull back the curtain" of your decisions with students, you can begin to explicitly teach them the steps of the decision-making process.

Step One: Identify the decision to be made. There are times when students do not even understand that they need to decide between two or more things. Those decisions may be actions or physical items. Not making a choice is also a decision. As teachers, we need to be explicit and make students aware of the choices that are before them.

Step Two: Gather information. In this step, we must gather all the information needed to make the best decision. This might mean contemplating our values and desires and researching a topic more deeply.

Step Three: Consider all the potential choices. While it is tempting to immediately dismiss some of the potential choices, it is important to look carefully at all of them. Consider what the alternatives are, including a variety of action steps (or none at all) that could be taken. Think through the potential consequences of each choice before you. This is a challenging step for students, as they may not have the foresight or experience to think of potential consequences for various actions.

Step Four: Decide and take action. Once you have considered the various possibilities and the consequences of each option, it is time to decide and take action.

Step Five: Consider the outcomes and consequences of the decision. Once action has been taken, reflect on the effectiveness of the action and whether it led to the desired outcomes. This is often a forgotten step for many people but is important to help them become aware of how their decisions potentially affected others and their own circumstances.

In addition to real-world decisions, we can also have students analyze decisions made by characters in literature or people in history. This gives students a more objective platform to discuss the decision-making process and consider how specific choices affect the outcome. Ultimately, students should be able to identify decisions they make at school and how those decisions affect them and their learning. The decisions students make help them in terms of the other SEL competencies, including self-management and relationship skills. Students need to learn that the decisions they make affect others, too. While this may seem abstract to students at first, the more they practice, the easier it will become.

Developing Student Autonomy

To self-manage effectively, students need to make good decisions. Helping students learn to make good decisions begins with presenting students with choices related to their learning. In many classrooms, students can focus only on the activity, task, or content that the teacher has designed. Other activities or ways to learn information and concepts are not offered and even are expressly forbidden in some cases. To build student autonomy and allow them to make responsible decisions, we must offer students choices as often and in as many contexts as possible. While this may seem daunting, consider the following types of autonomy and choices we can build into our instruction to help build student autonomy over time.

Organizational Autonomy

In organizational autonomy, students make decisions about common topics associated with classroom management so that they are less likely to need the teacher to give specific solutions or use directives. Students can give feedback on and help determine a variety of aspects of the classroom, including the following:

- Seating arrangements
- Group members
- Classroom rules and expectations

Student Choice in Seating Arrangements

There has been significant discussion and research (Barrett et al. 2013) regarding flexible seating in the classroom. Flexible seating involves providing options for students in terms of where they sit and the type of seating available. It moves away from the traditional school desks as the sole seating option and offers other seating options, such as cushions, chairs, couches, balls, and stools, for students to choose from.

Flexible seating has multiple benefits, including providing movement opportunities for students, more comfort, and community building and collaboration opportunities. The key words are *student choice*. The purpose is to have students make responsible decisions for their learning and choose seats that will help them learn. The focus of flexible seating should always be on enhancing engagement and learning. The purpose is not to sit comfortably with friends and disengage from the learning. The purpose is just the opposite, in fact: to sit comfortably to focus and stay engaged, thus enhancing learning.

When students have a choice of where to sit, they are empowered to control their own environments to focus and learn more effectively. Students should choose seats that they find comfortable at the time, which may mean changing seats throughout the day, depending on the situation and the learning task. It may feel comfortable to work at a desk for a writing assignment but more comfortable to sit on the floor on a cushion for a reading assignment. Small-group discussions might take place while sitting on stools in a circle.

Building choice into the seating arrangement also builds community, as students are not locked into one specific space that is "theirs"; rather, all students share all the seating options in the classroom. Students may find that they prefer one specific seating option and may want to stay there all the time. However, flexible seating should encourage opportunities for all students to use the various seating options. This might involve setting up a rotation schedule for students, as well as adjusting the options for students over time, building in more of the most popular seating options.

Finally, a discussion of rules and norms of behavior in implementing flexible seating is critical, as making responsible decisions will keep students safe and enhance the learning experience. Students should know that you will move them if they are not making appropriate decisions.

Student Choice in Group Members

Allowing students to choose who they work with at various points in the school day can seem overwhelming and may even cause you some anxiety. Will students choose only their friends? Will they get off task? Will the classroom get too noisy? Will there be a student who no one wants to work with?

Although these concerns are valid, building autonomy for students to choose whom they will work with, be it through flexible seating opportunities or in group formation, is another aspect of providing organizational autonomy. However, you don't have to allow students to choose their group members every time. It is important to consider when it is appropriate to have students choose the people they will work with and when you will choose and assign partners or small groups. For longer-term projects, for example, it may benefit students to work with people of their choice, especially if they have had experience working with others and know whom they work well with. In other cases, it may be better for you to assign groups, allowing students to gain experience working with different students or groups of students. Throughout the instructional day, students should have the opportunity to work with a wide variety of students, especially for short-term conversations or assignments. As students get to know one another, they will learn to make responsible decisions when it comes to choosing whom they will work with.

Student Choice in Classroom Rules and Expectations

Working with students to create behavioral expectations and rules is a tried-and-true way to build buy-in and ownership in how the classroom runs. Classroom rules should involve discussing both your expectations and students' expectations to best meet their needs and help them learn.

A great way to begin is by having students write or draw their ideas about the most important elements of a safe and respectful classroom. Next, work to create a list of potential rules or expectations. This can be done in numerous ways, including having students get together in small groups to create what their top three rules or expectations for classroom behavior should be. A classroom discussion can also be conducted; just be sure that as many students as possible are able to voice their opinions and provide input. Even though there will likely be more ideas than needed, having a larger list will help with the next step. Once a list has been made, students should come to a consensus on which rules should be implemented through a class, group, or anonymous vote. It is best to limit the final number of rules or expectations to three to five.

It can be helpful to also phrase the rules or expectations in a positive way so that students are clear as to what they *should* be doing, as opposed to what they *should not* be doing. For example, you might have "Listen respectfully" rather than "Don't talk while others are talking." Leading students through a discussion of how to reframe rules into positive language and expectations helps clarify the expectations.

The purpose of this exercise is not only to create classroom rules or expectations but also to build responsible decision-making skills. By choosing the expectations that will govern their classroom, students have begun their journeys of making responsible decisions. This is a complicated task, and students will need guidance. But by leading students through this process, you are building critical skills that will benefit them, and you, throughout the school year.

Procedural Autonomy

Procedural autonomy involves students making decisions in terms of the classroom procedures, including having students choose different materials they can use for projects and assignments, as well as the formats and media for formative and summative assessments.

Student Choice of Materials

Choosing materials for learning has traditionally been the job of the teacher. In fact, students often are not even aware of what materials are available to them to help them learn and grow in the different content areas. While having access to many different materials can potentially be a distraction for students, knowing what their options are and what they can use to help them learn is a powerful tool for developing autonomy.

Many teachers have students use graphic organizers for a variety of instructional purposes, including brainstorming, planning for writing, comparing and contrasting, or showing cause and effect. The use of graphic organizers, however, can be limited to the teacher demonstrating the use of the graphic for instructional purposes or having students use only one type of graphic organizer for assignments.

To build in responsible decision-making, you can share a variety of graphic organizers or planning tools with students over time, and then have students decide which tool is best for a particular assignment.

Consider the following scenario: You are assigning an informational or informative writing task to students. They have been studying the content for a few weeks and have a variety of sources to choose from. They need to take the information they have learned and create a piece of writing that integrates information from those sources.

As students begin the planning process, you share several options for them to plan their writing assignments. Each student must provide a planning tool wherein they share the ideas they will build into their writing. But students can decide on one of several tools, including the following:

A grid that shows the examples and features of the topic being studied:

Example	Characteristic A	Characteristic B
Example 1	▸ Specifics ▸ Specifics ▸ Specifics	▸ Specifics ▸ Specifics ▸ Specifics
Example 2	▸ Specifics ▸ Specifics ▸ Specifics	▸ Specifics ▸ Specifics ▸ Specifics
Example 3	▸ Specifics ▸ Specifics ▸ Specifics	▸ Specifics ▸ Specifics ▸ Specifics

A web diagram:

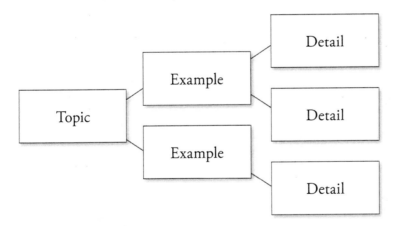

An outline:

1. Example

   a. Detail

   b. Detail

   c. Detail

A sketch or drawing:

Topic: Organisms of the Kelp Forest

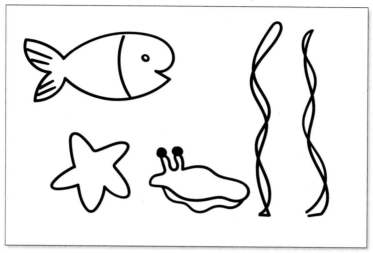

Once students have learned about the various options they have for planning, they decide which planning tools will serve them best for the task at hand and use them to complete the assignment.

Student Choice to Demonstrate Competence

Allowing students to choose how they will demonstrate competence and learning is another great way to build in procedural autonomy and promote responsible decision-making. Similar to having students choose graphic organizers, providing choices in formative and summative assessments allows students to play on their strengths and demonstrate what they know in a way that is comfortable for them.

Choice boards are one tool students can use to demonstrate competence. To create and share a choice board with students, consider the objectives for the lesson or unit and what students need to know and be able to do based on learning. Then brainstorm ideas for how students can demonstrate their knowledge in a way that is appropriate for their grade level. Try to build activities that relate to a variety of learning modalities, including visual, kinesthetic, auditory, and reading/writing, and consider the resources and materials available to students. Share the choice board with students, and have them choose the way they want to demonstrate their learning. To reinforce responsible decision-making, have students justify why they chose a specific way to demonstrate their knowledge. The generic choice board in figure 5.1 can be used as an example and modified based on the grade level and content students are learning. For additional sample choice boards, refer to the Digital Resources.

Figure 5.1. Sample Choice Board

Write and illustrate a picture book.	Create an online interactive illustration or drawing.	Make a time line.
Write an advertisement.	Create a screencast.	Write a song.
Design a tableau and demonstrate it live, via video, or take a picture.	Develop a board game.	Create a survey and administer it.

Cognitive Autonomy

Cognitive autonomy refers to a person's ability to think independently and have independent attitudes, values, and beliefs. When children develop cognitive autonomy, they are able to evaluate their own thinking, find multiple solutions to problems using creativity and innovation, justify those solutions, and receive feedback from you and their peers. Cognitive autonomy and responsible decision-making go hand in hand. As students develop cognitive autonomy, they are better able to not only make informed decisions but also evaluate the effectiveness of those decisions and the consequences.

In developing cognitive autonomy, students should have the opportunity to decide what they would like to learn, as well as to reflect on the learning process and what works for their learning styles. To develop students' cognitive autonomy skills, help students learn to do the following:

- Find multiple solutions to problems
- Reflect on their learning and what benefits them
- Give and receive feedback

Finding Multiple Solutions to Problems

Problem-solving is a key life skill that will benefit students for the rest of their lives. Yet in the classroom, some students may be presented with one particular way of solving a problem and not given alternatives or asked to develop additional strategies or solutions to problems. In many classrooms, the typical instructional pattern is to state either a current or past problem and tell students what the solution to the problem is. Students are then expected to implement the solution.

Classroom management is one area where this scenario plays out. Students who misbehave or cause a disruption, for example, are instructed to stop or told to do something different. These disruptions, however, provide opportunities for students to find their own solutions to the problems. Based on the classroom rules and expectations, for example, students can also have potential solutions for those not following the expectations. Note that this does not mean that students give consequences or punishments to one another; rather, they seek solutions or alternatives for their classmates when they are being disruptive.

Students can also explore ways to solve problems through content. It is common in mathematics for students to look at different ways to solve equations. In science, students may determine a variety of ways to test a hypothesis. In social studies, students may look at many potential solutions around a topic in history or a current event. In language arts, students might explore how a particular character could resolve a problem or issue they are facing. Look for opportunities for students to analyze and discuss multiple ways to solve problems, as well as which tool or action would be the best choice and why they think so.

Reflecting on Learning

Reflection is a powerful tool for teachers and students alike. It provides the opportunity to consider what works in teaching and learning and how the information will benefit us. When students reflect on learning and what is helpful and useful for them as learners, they build cognitive autonomy as they think through the benefits of both the learning process and the newly acquired information. Opportunities for reflection can be built in almost any time by providing students with information about the relevance of the content, such as how one concept relates to different careers or to other information being learned or how it may be used in the future. By considering this information, students can make important decisions about their learning and what they want to learn in the future.

Giving and Receiving Feedback

The ability to give solid feedback and to receive feedback is another key aspect of cognitive autonomy that will benefit students in the long-term. To provide effective feedback, students need to first know what to look for and then decide what they will and will not comment on. From there, they will need to provide specific feedback that is helpful to the other student. Finally, the person receiving the feedback should articulate their actions (or nonactions) based on the feedback they received. Figure 5.2 depicts the feedback process. The gray boxes show the actions of the person giving the feedback. The white boxes show the actions of the person receiving the feedback.

Competency Connections

Reflection on learning is a form of metacognition. Metacognition helps students be more self-aware as they consider how they best learn and what they are interested in. Asking students metacognitive reflection questions, such as "What helped you learn?" and "How might this information benefit you in the future?" builds both personal reflection and metacognition.

Figure 5.2. The Feedback Process

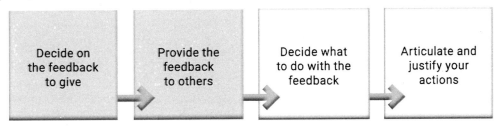

| Decide on the feedback to give | Provide the feedback to others | Decide what to do with the feedback | Articulate and justify your actions |

Decide on the feedback to give: The first step starts with specific criteria as determined in the standards, potentially with input from students about what may need to change. For example, you can provide students with a rubric that shows lesson specifications that a task will be evaluated on. Then students can discuss which areas will be focused on at a given time before providing feedback.

Provide the feedback to others: When giving feedback, students should start with and build on the positive aspects of the assignment. In other words, do not begin with phrases such as "Can I give you some feedback?" as this immediately puts up defense mechanisms in people. When students share compliments or strengths first, they are building a positive rapport with the other student and are more likely to be able to receive the corrective feedback that comes next.

After providing some positive aspects of the assignment, provide feedback on areas that need adjustment. In this step, have students practice using suggestive words, such as *option*, *consider*, and *possible*. These words make the feedback more likely to be heard and taken for what they are: suggestions. As students share their suggestions, the person receiving the feedback should record the comments and notes on what the suggestions entailed. The student receiving the feedback can then choose which, if any, suggestions to consider changing.

Another important aspect of giving and getting feedback is to state instructions as instructions and not as suggestions. In other words, if the assignment requires students to include three pieces of evidence from a text and the writer only includes two, explicitly state that one piece of evidence is missing and that they have not met the requirements. While the author may decide to not include the additional evidence, they are doing so knowing that this feedback was about an instruction, not a suggestion.

Decide what to do with the feedback: After getting feedback, it is important to teach students to be objective and decide how, or if, they will incorporate the feedback they were given. Provide students the opportunity to reflect on their decision-making process here. They should consider their decisions, act on the feedback or not, and consider the consequences of their decisions. Once they have evaluated the consequences and implemented any feedback, they can consider how the actions or inactions have changed or improved the assignment.

Articulate and justify your actions: Last, have students articulate the suggestions and solutions that they were offered and whether they took the suggestions. Students should then justify their actions/inactions based on the feedback received. This reflection is important as they share their decision-making process. When students reflect on the effectiveness of their decisions, they can apply decision-making in other situations.

Decision-Making in Action

A variety of strategies can be used to teach students responsible decision-making. These strategies help students improve decision-making skills over time. Even having students make small decisions on a daily basis builds their autonomy and decision-making capabilities. When students have choices, it builds engagement. When students are only encouraged to follow the precise directions, we are reinforcing compliance as opposed to decision-making. The following strategies can be adapted for a variety of grade levels and used in different content areas.

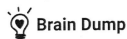

Brain Dump

This strategy involves students brainstorming all ideas, solutions, or outcomes for decisions they are considering. It is critical that Brain Dump begins with one simple ground rule: all ideas will be welcomed and considered. For students to be successful in brainstorming, they must break the cycle of negative personal feedback they may tell themselves, wherein they don't share ideas out of fear of the ideas being rejected. To combat this, students can begin brainstorming on topics that have low risk, such as possible characters for a story. This strategy is about quantity, not quality. When students can write many ideas, there is a higher likelihood that an idea or ideas will come to fruition.

Similarities, Differences, and Connections

To make a responsible decision, students need information. Depending on the decision, students can think through their choices. By considering the similarities, differences, and connections between choices, students can begin to see how the choices converge and diverge to best make a solid decision. Begin by teaching students the language they need to think through the similarities, differences, and connections between choices. Using academic language helps bridge social-emotional learning with content-area instruction. Consider the following words and sentence frames that can be used as students analyze their decisions. Have students engage in discussions about their choices, characters' choices from books or novels, or decisions made in history.

Compare-and-Contrast Signal Words

like	but	yet	is the same as
unlike	both	are similar because	on the other hand
however	are the same/ different because	_____er/_____est	_____er than

Continued

have in common	difference between	just like/as	a distinction between
in contrast	as opposed to	compared to	share common attributes
synonymous with	each is	by comparison	whereas

Sample Sentence Frames

▸ Both are/are able to/have/can _____.

▸ _____ and _____ are similar because they are both _____.

▸ _____ and _____ are different because _____ is _____ and _____ is _____.

▸ Although _____ and _____ have some similar characteristics, they are very different because _____.

▸ The majority of _____ are _____, while _____ are _____.

▸ The differences/similarities between _____ and _____ are _____.

▸ The _____ and _____ are similar in that _____.

▸ While _____ and _____ are both _____, there are several major differences between them.

▸ The most noticeable/notable difference is that _____ has _____, whereas _____ has _____.

▸ The primary distinction between _____ and _____ can be described as _____.

Paragraph Frames for Comparing and Contrasting

▸ _____ and _____ are similar in a variety of ways. They both _____. They also are similar in that _____. Moreover, each _____. Because of these similarities, we can _____.

▸ However, _____ and _____ differ in several ways. For example, _____, whereas _____. In addition, _____ is _____, but _____ is _____. Furthermore, _____ is _____, different from _____, which is _____. These differences help us see _____.

💡 Visual Decision-Making

Analyzing the consequences or outcomes of a decision can be an abstract concept for students. Using the Visual Decision-Making strategy, students explore possible consequences of decisions through graphic organizers. Figure 5.3 shows several graphic organizers and how they can be used to help students visualize the outcomes of decisions.

Figure 5.3. Graphic Organizers for Decision-Making

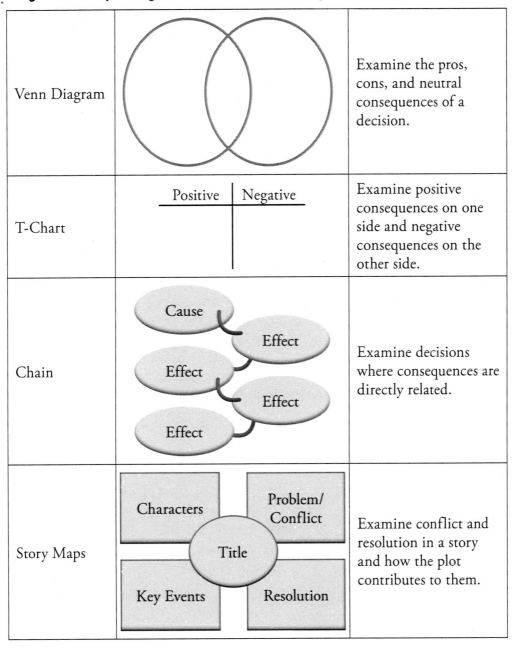

Venn Diagram		Examine the pros, cons, and neutral consequences of a decision.
T-Chart	Positive / Negative	Examine positive consequences on one side and negative consequences on the other side.
Chain	Cause, Effect, Effect, Effect, Effect	Examine decisions where consequences are directly related.
Story Maps	Characters, Problem/Conflict, Title, Key Events, Resolution	Examine conflict and resolution in a story and how the plot contributes to them.

Teaching students words and phrases that signal a cause-and-effect relationship builds their academic language and supports discussion of their visual decision-making maps. The following list includes some examples of this type of vocabulary.

if _____, then _____	when (cause), then (effect)	which in turn
as a result (of)	even if _____, would	the fact that
consequently	accordingly	because
due to	once _____, _____	therefore
leads me to believe	for this reason	since
subsequently	after (cause), then (effect)	one reason for
so	it follows	leads/led to

Role-Playing

Once the decisions and their effects or consequences are identified, students can role-play what those decisions and the results might look like. This concept can be linked to different subject areas as well, including social studies, language arts, science, or mathematics. Students can do this in pairs or small groups and play the parts of different people making the same or different decisions.

Through role-play, students can gain differing perspectives on how particular decisions may change the consequences. By role-playing, students can make abstract consequences more concrete.

The SWOT Analysis

The SWOT Analysis (figure 5.4) is a tool that students can use to consider decisions. *SWOT* stands for *strengths*, *weaknesses*, *opportunities*, and *threats*. Students can discuss and write about each area as it relates to a particular decision.

- ▶ **Strengths:** What are the positive aspects of this decision? What strengths or benefits will result from this decision?
- ▶ **Weaknesses:** What are the costs of this decision? What are the negative aspects?

▶ **Opportunities:** What new doors might open? What opportunities are there based on the decision?

▶ **Threats:** What can get in the way of success? What obstacles might you face?

Figure 5.4.

SWOT Analysis	
Describe the decision:	
Strengths	
Weaknesses	
Opportunities	
Threats	

 ## The SODAS Method

SODAS stands for *situation, options, disadvantages, advantages,* and *solution.* Students consider each of the following areas as they analyze their decisions. SODAS can also be used to consider decisions made by people in history or characters in stories or novels.

Situation: Describe the situation in detail. What is happening? What is the context in which it is happening?

Options: What options are there? Which options are realistic, and which options are not as realistic?

Disadvantages: What are the disadvantages of each decision? What might be the negative consequences of each option?

Advantages: What are the advantages of each decision? What might be the positive consequences of each option?

Solution: Based on what you have considered, make a decision that will lead to the best solution possible. The solution may not be perfect or ideal but is the best possible solution given the situation, options, advantages, and disadvantages.

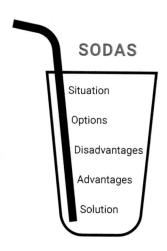

 Would You Rather. . .?

A fun and engaging game to play with students is "Would You Rather...?" In this game, often played in pairs, students must consider specific sets of choices. They then discuss the pros and cons of their choices and ultimately make a decision. Of course, the decision does not need to be executed; rather, it is discussed. It can be fun to share strange or even ridiculous choices with students so that they can talk through the decisions and consequences. Here are a few examples. The Digital Resources contain additional questions on printable cards.

Would you rather...

- ▶ have a magic carpet or your own personal robot?
- ▶ see a fireworks display or go to a concert?
- ▶ fly a kite or ride a scooter?
- ▶ ride in a jet plane or on a train?
- ▶ never take another shower or never have to clip your toenails again?

Stop and Reflect

1. Consider your classroom and the opportunities students have to make decisions. In what ways can you provide additional opportunities for students to make responsible decisions in the classroom? What specific guidance and scaffolds will students need to practice this essential skill?

2. How does responsible decision-making involve the other SEL competencies, and how can you make that connection clear to students?

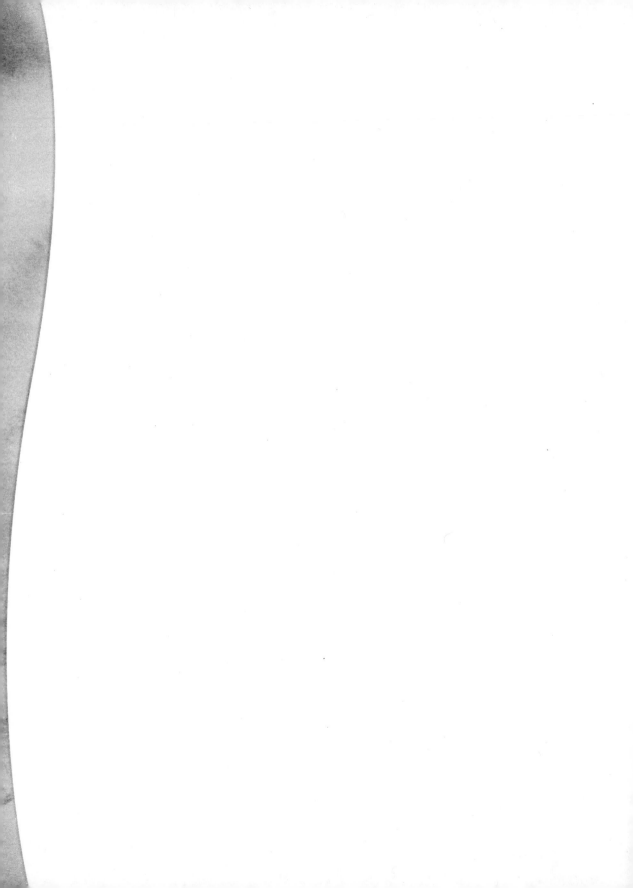

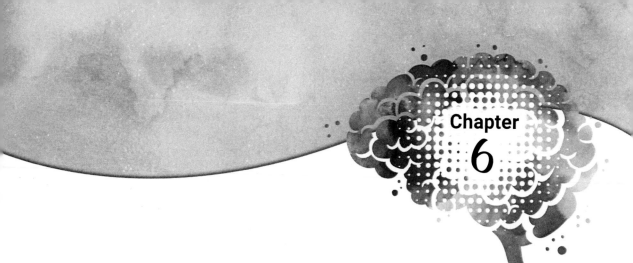

Putting It All Together

Social-emotional learning should be embedded in every aspect of education. The research shows the positive effects it has on students, but more than that, it is the morally and ethically right thing to do. You likely became an educator because you love children and want them to learn and grow up to be happy, healthy individuals who can accomplish anything they want in life. While having solid content knowledge is of critical importance, if people do not have the competencies outlined in this book, it will be extremely difficult for them to get there.

Implementing SEL lessons less frequently will not lead to students deeply understanding and practicing SEL. Building SEL competencies and skills will require focus throughout each and every day as we deepen our awareness of students, their well-being, and our own mental health.

How to Start

While the ultimate goal is to have SEL integrated into each aspect of the school day and beyond so that students internalize the competencies and skills outlined in this book, it is unrealistic to think we can all get there instantaneously. As you consider where to start, think of SEL implementation as a road map.

Consider what you are already doing. Think about which competencies you already have in place that may just need to be extended or strengthened and which come naturally to you. This is an excellent place to start. Given that you already feel comfortable with a particular competency, it will be easier to build on that foundation. Look for additional strategies you can use in the classroom, and consider where in your lessons and in your day you might build in those skills.

Consider a specific time of day or subject area that is a natural fit for SEL integration. You may find that starting the day with a focus on SEL and intentionally weaving in some strategies will set the stage for the rest of the day and help you integrate skills more frequently. Similarly, you may find that the end of the day is a great time to integrate SEL more intentionally, as it helps wrap up the day in a way that focuses on well-being as students head home. Or you may find that a subject area lends itself well to the integration of SEL competencies and skills. Whatever the scenario, choose a time and focus that work for you, and get started!

Once you have established a competency that feels natural, consider one that will be a challenge to integrate and commit to putting that in action. Perhaps it is a competency that you feel you need to strengthen for yourself or one that you do not feel as comfortable teaching. Starting with at least one challenging aspect right away can increase momentum. Start small with a manageable challenge and continue to build on it as it becomes a part of your teaching practice.

The same practice can be done in terms of times of day or subject areas. Choose a time of day in which students have some challenges and the integration of SEL would benefit them. Or you might consider that a particular subject area does not lend itself easily to integration of SEL. Look at a particular lesson plan or unit and carefully consider opportunities to build in some strategies, skills, and concepts.

I recommend implementing this strategy for one key reason. Generally, if we start with the practices that we feel comfortable with or that seem easy to do, we may never get to the challenging ones. If we only focus on areas that are especially challenging, we may feel discouraged and may not continue. By focusing on both easy and more challenging aspects of SEL integration, we will have a more successful integration of all aspects of SEL more frequently throughout the day.

Into, Through, and Beyond: An SEL Framework for Success

As you consider implementation of SEL in your classroom, in your school, or in your district, use the Into, Through, and Beyond framework to ground your thinking and prepare for success (see figure 6.1). Each step involves planning, action, and reflection. As you build on your current skills, add new strategies, and consider their effectiveness and their effect on your students, SEL will become a more natural part of who you are and how you teach. With intentionality, you will continue to build a better world, helping students gain the skills they will need to lead happy and productive lives.

Figure 6.1. The Into, Through, and Beyond SEL Framework Model

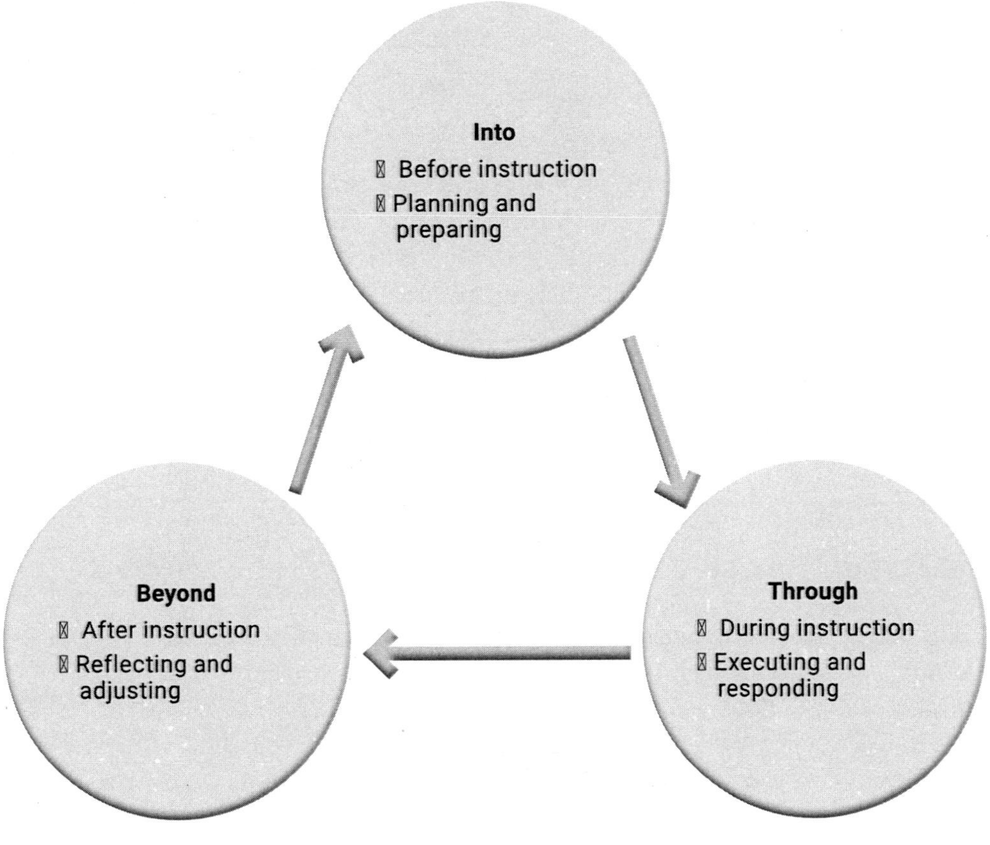

Into
- Before instruction
- Planning and preparing

Through
- During instruction
- Executing and responding

Beyond
- After instruction
- Reflecting and adjusting

The Into, Through, and Beyond framework is recursive in nature. We move through the process continually planning, teaching, and implementing strategies and skills that will help us throughout our lives. The beginning of the process is linear—as you move through the phases, you may begin planning what is next, continue to practice and adjust based on successes and setbacks, and look for ways to develop skills with students.

The Into Phase

The "into" phase of the framework includes planning and preparation. It is the phase prior to instruction—everything you do to get ready to teach, whether it's the start of a new lesson, a new unit, or a new school year. Take stock of the strategies and techniques you are currently using to build instruction in the five SEL competencies. How are you already demonstrating and teaching these competencies? Which have worked well? Continue building on those strengths. Which areas need additional emphasis? What specific competencies do students and the community need? Choose a few strategies that you think will help meet those needs and teach them.

Consider your own readiness as well as students' readiness, and which strategies will help set the stage for deeper implementation of the SEL competencies. Also think about where you are in terms of the school year, the unit of study, and the lessons you will be providing. It may make more sense to focus on one specific competency if you are starting the school year, such as relationship building, before you deeply dive into the other competencies. It may be that a particular unit of study you are focusing on lends itself to one of the competencies, such as responsible decision-making. Your needs, students' needs, and the content you are teaching may intersect to help you plan where to start or what your next steps will be.

The Through Phase

This phase is everything that happens during instruction. It's how we put our planning into action by integrating SEL instruction into our lessons, our daily routines, and our classroom environment.

Sometimes, as we implement a new strategy or technique, we do not get the immediate results we are looking for. That can lead us to say to ourselves, "This doesn't work." However, it may be that we have not given the strategy enough time to be internalized by students, or we have not yet become comfortable enough with the strategy to make it a natural part of our teaching. As you teach the competencies, use a variety of strategies that help you and your students deeply internalize and practice the competences. Look for ways to explicitly and intentionally teach and practice the SEL competencies and ways to informally and consistently remind students of these skills. As with any concept or skill, we should use the teach-model-practice-apply routine. Teach students the concept or skill explicitly. Students should know what the competency or skill is, why it is important, and how to do it or demonstrate it. Then model the skill for students. This can and should be done when teaching the skill but also throughout each day of instruction. Point out how you are demonstrating the skill. After modeling, have students practice the skill. This can be done through an activity so that students are practicing outside of a context that may be more emotionally charged. Finally, continually encourage students to apply the skill throughout the days and weeks ahead, as situations arise that allow them to weave the skill and competency into their lives.

This phase also includes how we react in the moment and respond to students from both an academic and an SEL perspective. Because instruction rarely goes *exactly* as we plan, it's important to continue to build your toolkit of SEL strategies so that you can respond appropriately and support students with their own social-emotional learning development.

The Beyond Phase

As we lean into implementation, we will need to continually reflect on the effectiveness of our practice and look at next steps in terms of implementation and internalization of the SEL competencies and skills. Continually reflect on where to go next. How can we infuse the strategies and skills in all aspects of our lives? How can we build on the skills we are learning? Which students do you need to follow up with, and what is the best way to do this?

Remember that as a teacher, you are not necessarily a mental health professional. It may be that some students will need additional support beyond the scope of SEL competencies and skills in the classroom. Ask yourself, *Which students may need additional support beyond what I can provide in the classroom? Who can I share my concerns or questions with? A counselor or administrator? How and when should I express concern or share information with parents?*

The WOOP Strategy

The WOOP Strategy, developed by Gabriele Oettingen (2015), is a research-based method to develop motivation and change habits. The strategy contains four steps, outlined by the acronym *WOOP*, which stands for *wish, outcome, obstacles, plan*. The WOOP Strategy is designed to help students set a goal or a wish to accomplish and determine how to fulfill it. This strategy can be used to help you and students accomplish goals within any of the competencies.

> **Wish:** Develop a goal or a wish to accomplish. The goal should be feasible and realistic.

> **Outcome:** Envision what the future will look like once the goal or wish is met.

> **Obstacles:** Identify the challenges and obstacles that will need to be confronted or overcome. Determine the most critical obstacle.

> **Plan:** Plan how to overcome the identified obstacles. Consider the actions needed to overcome those obstacles.

Teaching the WOOP Strategy

Wish

Goal setting can be challenging for students, as they may want to set goals that are unrealistic or unrelated to education. While the strategy can be used for any goal, begin by focusing on goals related to the classroom, including social, behavioral, and academic goals, as appropriate. Goal-setting activities can be scaffolded for students based on their grade and maturity level, using a variety of activities.

For example, begin by sharing your sample wishes or goals with students. These might be wishes or goals that you have developed for yourself, examples you have developed for students, or examples from previous students you have worked with. Then discuss the purpose of the goals and why they are realistic.

To make the learning hands-on, have some goals printed and cut into strips. These can be the examples you shared, goals that have been discussed from stories or novels, or goals that students have begun developing for themselves. In pairs or small groups, have students sort the goals based on differing criteria. For example, you might have students sort the goals into realistic versus unrealistic and discuss why a goal falls under the chosen category.

From there, students write or design their own wishes or goals. Begin with shorter-term goals so that students can analyze their levels of success or what needs to be accomplished to achieve the goal. If a goal is too long-term, students may get discouraged and not want to continue working toward meeting the goal.

Outcome

As in the wish stage of this strategy, students may struggle knowing what the future will look like when their goals are accomplished. This is true for people of all ages. However, students can be guided through the process to help them see what the outcome of their goals will look like.

Book and story analysis is one way to begin this process. Once the goal has been set, the outcome can be analyzed. Did the outcome match what the person had envisioned? What helped make the goal a reality, or what hindered the process? This analysis helps students dig in deeper to the reading and consider potential outcomes.

Arts integration can be used to help students envision their goals. Through drawing and sketching, students can represent what the physical or emotional outcomes of their goals will be. For example, what will the project look like if the goal is attained? Or how will attaining the goal make students feel? Students can represent these outcomes visually as a way to see the outcome and help make it more concrete.

Group brainstorming is another useful activity, as others' ideas can help spark potential outcomes. Have students get as many ideas on paper as possible in a given time frame, without judgment. This works well when the time frame is short and allows students to not worry about ridicule, allowing creativity to flow. Sometimes the ideas that first seem ridiculous end up being the most innovative and interesting.

Obstacles

The next step is to determine the obstacles that can make the goal or wish more challenging to accomplish. To teach students about potential obstacles, take them through a scenario of a wish or goal, and share with them the obstacles that may come into play. This may be as simple as sharing a short journey around the classroom and the obstacles that may be encountered when trying to get from one point to another. More complex wishes and goals and their obstacles can also be shared depending on students' ages and grade levels.

From there, have students brainstorm some wishes or goals as a class, and brainstorm the potential obstacles that may need overcoming to accomplish these goals. It is important to help students differentiate between task-oriented and personal obstacles, as these may be dealt with differently. Personal obstacles can be motivation levels, unhelpful habits, debilitating emotions, or limiting beliefs. These are very helpful to identify as part of the self-management process but do not necessarily need to be shared publicly. Task-oriented obstacles are directly related to the task. These are appropriate to share publicly and brainstorm, as students can brainstorm potential solutions or ways to overcome or eliminate these obstacles.

Plan

The final step in the WOOP Strategy is to plan. Again, it is important to model the planning process. Planning can take many forms, including when and how to get started, how to continue moving forward, and how to deal with potential obstacles. Share with students any tools that you use to plan when considering your wishes and goals.

Graphic organizers are effective tools for planning. Students can consider times and places to work toward their wishes and goals and the necessary materials and conditions that will make their work more productive. Students can also brainstorm *if/then* statements, both orally and in writing, to plan for the obstacles that may come into play as they work toward meeting their wishes and goals. Figure 6.2 shows a sample WOOP Strategy graphic organizer.

Figure 6.2. WOOP Strategy Graphic Organizer

| Wish: | Materials: |
| | Conditions: |

| If/Then Statement: | |

| Outcome: | Materials: |
| | Conditions: |

| If/Then Statement: | |

| Obstacle: | Materials: |
| | Conditions: |

| If/Then Statement: | |

| Plan: | Materials: |
| | Conditions: |

| If/Then Statement: | |

School-Wide Implementation of SEL

"I've learned that people will forget what you said, people will forget what you did, but people will never forget how you made them feel."
—Maya Angelou

While one teacher can make the difference in the life of a student, another person can unknowingly or inadvertently cause setbacks in a student's social-emotional growth. Each of us plays a role in positively affecting students. When SEL is incorporated across grade levels, in an entire school, or throughout the district, we build on student success from multiple angles and over the course of time.

As with any standard or skill, students will need continual practice as they get older and more mature and as life and circumstances get more complicated. Consider, for example, the study of habitats and organisms in science, the study of character development in language arts, or the study of place value in mathematics. As students progress through the years, these topics become more complex, and students learn more and more about the complexities that exist within the topics. Social-emotional skills are no different; they build on each other, and students need practice and instruction throughout the grade levels to be successful. Here is an example:

Standard: Identify and manage one's emotions and behavior.

Kindergarten: Identify feelings in characters in stories and in oneself.

5th Grade: Use specific strategies to manage one's own emotions and be self-reflective.

12th Grade: Understand how one's emotions affect others, and find community resources to effectively self-manage.

Incorporating SEL at a school-wide level also helps build a strong community and a culture of respect, understanding, and learning in a school. As students learn how to regulate and manage their emotions, they are better able to make good decisions for their learning and thereby help build a classroom community that promotes learning. Additionally, as students develop social awareness and take others' perspectives into account, they build a culture of respect and empathy.

As this community of respect and learning is built, students communicate more effectively with one another, develop positive working relationships, and are able to work collaboratively toward learning goals. These skills, of course, are not built overnight, nor are they perfected when practiced in only one classroom over the course of one year. In a school-wide approach, students can begin learning skills in kindergarten and continue practicing the skills throughout their education.

School Culture

School culture has a strong impact on social-emotional learning, and relationships are what drive the culture of a school. Through deeper connections, we are able to embody and teach the SEL competencies and help create a culture of caring and support in schools. Consider the culture at your school. Are the teachers, staff, and administration happy? Is it common for the adults in the building to smile at one another and students? Do people stop to greet one another and chat in the hallways? Are people in staff meetings open, respectful, and interested in what others have to say? The culture of the staff, including the way the adults relate to one another, will have a major impact on students' culture and on implementation of social-emotional learning in the school and classroom.

Building Relationships

Building and fostering relationships is perhaps one of the best ways we can strengthen school culture to increase SEL practices. Several types of relationships exist in schools; each requires attention to create a school culture that truly integrates SEL practices.

Adult Relationships

Relationships among adults are critical and have a huge influence on the culture of the school. In schools with strong social-emotional learning, the adults do the following:

> ▸ **Collaborate on their practice.** They share ideas with one another through formal and informal means, including in staff meetings, in professional learning communities, and through informal discussions and communications.
>
> ▸ **Celebrate one another.** They share accomplishments and give shout-outs and compliments to one another.

▸ **Address conflicts through solution-based means.** When disagreements, issues, and problems arise, they deal with them in ways that move toward solutions that everyone can support.

Adult–Student Relationships

Each student in the school should be known by at least one adult. That means that the adult not only knows the student's name but also knows something about the student, the adult has had multiple interactions with the student inside and outside of the classroom, and both parties treat each other with mutual respect. Developing deep relationships between adults and students requires the following:

▸ Students know that the adults care about them.

▸ Adults notice students and acknowledge their feelings. They notice when students are not themselves and check in with students.

▸ Adults engage students through their relationships with them, rather than through the content.

▸ Students feel comfortable approaching adults with concerns, issues, and problems, regardless of the severity.

Student–Student Relationships

Deep, meaningful collaboration among students will help build strong relationships. Collaboration does not focus exclusively on the end product but rather focuses on how students work together. For deep collaboration to work, students should do the following:

▸ Have roles that they are assigned, with individual input and accountability built in

▸ Provide constructive feedback to one another in ways that are helpful, specific, and kind

▸ Have the ability to work with other students, including students they like and get along well with and students they do not necessarily get along with

As discussed in the chapter on relationship skills, relationships among people can be fostered in many ways. To develop a deeper SEL culture within the school, be intentional about how you are building and fostering relationships with and among your colleagues and with and among students.

Addressing Self-Care

Let's face it: teaching is a difficult job. We are asked to focus on seemingly endless topics, skills, initiatives, requirements, challenges, and on and on. It can feel overwhelming and stressful. The most successful people in life are those who strike a balance between their professional and personal lives and are able to deal with stresses as they face them. Of course, by successful I do not mean only people who are financially successful. Rather, these people have found fulfillment in their work and have found a way to be healthy, happy individuals.

As teachers, we all need to find ways to care for ourselves. If we don't, we will not be able to care for those in our charge. Learning about and helping address the trauma students have faced is traumatic in and of itself. We must find ways to rejuvenate and release the stress and anxiety that can come with our profession. While each person is different, we can use a number of simple self-care strategies to help create balance and well-being. The following are just a few of the many strategies you might consider.

A friend once told me that taking time to do self-care activities sometimes made her even more stressed, as it meant she was not getting the "to-do" list done, which felt overwhelming. I sometimes feel the same way; when there is so much to do, how can I possibly take time to take care of myself? In these instances, start small. Take a few minutes here and there so that you can refocus and calm your brain and nerves for a few moments before tackling the next item on the to-do list.

Breathe Deeply: Even one minute of deep breathing helps oxygenate our brain and calm our bodies. Sit or stand comfortably, focus on your breath, fill your lungs to capacity, and release your breath completely several times. It is simple but effective!

Go for a Quick Walk: Getting outside when the weather allows provides us with fresh air, a change of scenery, and a bit of exercise. You don't have to take a long walk; a five-minute stroll around the school or around the block will help you refocus and rejuvenate!

Make a List with a Time Line: When you have a lot of tasks to complete, make a list. It can give great satisfaction to cross off items. By adding due dates, it gives you a better sense of what needs to be done and in what order. That can help you focus on what you want to accomplish at the moment.

Call or Chat with Someone You Love or Care About: This strategy relates back to relationship building. Our friends and family are great resources to help us feel better. Even a short call or chat to check on someone, ask them about their feelings related to something going on, or quickly catch up can help us feel more connected to others and lower our stress levels.

Plan a Vacation: While you might not have the time or money to go on a vacation, consider planning where you might go when and if you have the time and the money. Just the act of researching a place you would like to visit, looking at sites you might see, and considering why you would like to go there can boost excitement about the possibility of someday going there.

Humor Yourself: Find something that makes you laugh: a video clip, a comic strip, or a favorite comedian. It feels good to laugh, and a boost of positive emotions when we are feeling stress can help us better manage and release some of the stress we are feeling.

Listen to a Song You Love: Music is powerful; it can help us relax or boost our energy. Listening to music intently takes us away from our stressors or other areas of focus for a few minutes and brings us positive memories and feelings we associate with a particular song or artist.

While there are potentially hundreds of ways to practice self-care, choose ones that are manageable for you and that you can fit into your schedule. By practicing self-care on a regular basis, you will be able to better manage the challenges associated with our profession.

Final Thoughts

Whether you are just beginning your journey into SEL integration or have been studying and thinking about how you might intentionally weave SEL into your classroom practice, I am grateful that you have chosen this resource as a tool. Teachers have one of the most difficult jobs of all—caring for and educating our young people. Students must learn critical content knowledge and skills to be successful. To do that most effectively, and for students to lead the kinds of lives that will help make life better for everyone, it is critical to integrate and demonstrate SEL skills.

Integration of self-awareness, self-management, social awareness, relationship skills, and responsible decision-making is a lifelong process that takes thought, reflection, and action. The purpose of this book is to give you some actionable strategies that you can both integrate into your own life and share with students. As we practice and teach these strategies, they become a part of who we are and how we do things. As we deepen our awareness and implementation, the five competencies and the related skills become a way of life, leading to increased joy, resilience, deeper and more fulfilling relationships, and a way to fight injustice and make the world a better place for all.

Stop and Reflect

1. What was your primary motivation for reading this book? What needs are you hoping to address?

2. How deeply have you internalized the competencies? Which do you feel you demonstrate consistently and effectively already? Which do you feel you need to internalize more deeply?

3. What level of implementation are you aiming for as you plan to integrate SEL deeply and consistently? In your classroom? With your grade-level or subject-area colleagues? School-wide? District-wide?

4. Where will you start? Which competencies and strategies will you begin with, and why?

5. How will you share your successes and struggles, and with whom? Who can support you along the way?

6. How will you remember to practice self-care, and what strategies will you use to stay rejuvenated?

References Cited

Allen, Summer. 2018. *The Science of Gratitude*. Greater Good Science Center at UC Berkeley. https://ggsc.berkeley.edu/images/uploads/GGSC-JTF_White_Paper-Gratitude-FINAL.pdf.

Baker, Jean A., Sycarah Grant, and Larissa Morlock. 2008. "The Teacher-Student Relationship as a Developmental Context for Children with Internalizing or Externalizing Behavior Problems." *School Psychology Quarterly* 23 (1): 3–15.

Barker, Jane E., and Yuko Munakata. 2015. "Time Isn't of the Essence: Activating Goals Rather Than Imposing Delays Improves Inhibitory Control in Children." *Psychological Science* 26 (12): 1898–1908. https://www.ncbi.nlm.nih.gov/pmc/articles/PMC4679477/.

Barrett, Peter, Yufan Zhang, Joanne Moffat, and Khairy Kobbacy. 2013. "A Holistic, Multi-Level Analysis Identifying the Impact of Classroom Design on Pupils' Learning." *Building and Environment* 59: 678–89.

Bennett, Kathleen, and Dusana Dorjee. 2016. "The Impact of a Mindfulness-Based Stress Reduction Course (MBSR) on Well-Being and Academic Attainment of Sixth-Form Students." *Mindfulness* 7: 105–14. https://doi.org/10.1007/s12671-015-0430-7.

Brown, Philip, Michael W. Corrigan, and Ann Higgins-D'Alessandro. 2012. *Handbook of Prosocial Education*. Lanham, MD: Rowman & Littlefield.

Burke, Cassie Walker. 2018. "Three Out of Four Illinois Kids Aren't Ready for Kindergarten. Why That's a Problem." *Chalkbeat Chicago*, August 13, 2018. https://chalkbeat.org/posts/chicago/2018/08/13/three-out-of-four-illinois-kids-arent-ready-for-kindergarten/.

Center on the Social and Emotional Foundations for Early Learning. (n.d.) "Teaching Your Child to: Identify and Express Emotions." http://csefel.vanderbilt.edu/familytools/teaching_emotions.pdf.

Centers for Disease Control and Prevention, National Center for Injury Prevention and Control. n.d. *Web-based Injury Statistics Query and Reporting System (WISQARS)*. Accessed May 11, 2021. www.cdc.gov/injury/wisqars.

Chiesi, Harry L., George J. Spilich, and James F. Voss. 1979. "Acquisition of Domain-Related Information in Relation to High and Low Domain Knowledge." *Journal of Verbal Learning and Verbal Behavior* 18 (3): 257–73.

Collaborative for Academic, Social, and Emotional Learning (CASEL). 2021. "SEL: What Are the Core Competence Areas and Where Are They Promoted?" https://www.casel.org/sel -framework/.

Cook, Clayton R., Aria Fiat, Madeline Larson, Christopher Daikos, Tal Slemrod, Elizabeth A. Holland, Andrew J. Thayer, and Tyler Renshaw. 2018. "Positive Greetings at the Door: Evaluation of a Low-Cost, High-Yield Proactive Classroom Management Strategy." *Journal of Positive Behavior Interventions* 20 (3): 149–59.

Davidson, Richard J., Jon Kabat-Zinn, Jessica Schumacher, Melissa Rosenkranz, Daniel Muller, Saki F. Santorelli, Ferris Urbanowski, Anne Harrington, Katherine Bonus, and John F. Sheridan. 2003. "Alterations in Brain and Immune Function Produced by Mindfulness Meditation." *Psychosomatic Medicine* 65 (4): 564–70. https://ncbi.nlm.nih.gov/pubmed/12883106/.

Douglas, Ann. 2016. "Seven Surprising Facts about Emotions that Every Child Needs to Know." *Confident Parents Confident Kids* (blog post), September 22, 2016. https://confidentparentsconfidentkids.org/2016/09/22/seven-surprising-facts-about-emotions-that -every-child-needs-to-know/.

Dunlosky, John. 2013. "Strengthening the Student Toolbox." *American Educator* (Fall). https://www.aft.org/ae/fall2013/dunlosky.

Durlak, Joseph A., Roger P. Weissberg, Allison B. Dymnicki, Rebecca D. Taylor, and Kriston B. Schellinger. 2011. "The Impact of Enhancing Students' Social and Emotional Learning: A Meta-Analysis of School-Based Universal Interventions." *Child Development* 82 (1): 405–32.

Eisenberg, Nancy, Tracy L. Spinrad, and Natalie D. Eggum. 2010. "Emotion-Related Self-Regulation and Its Relation to Children's Maladjustment." *Annual Review of Clinical Psychology* 6: 495–525. https://doi.org/10.1146/annurev.clinpsy.121208.131208.

Ellis, Mesha L., Bahr Weiss, and John E. Lochman. 2009. "Executive Functions in Children: Associations with Aggressive Behavior and Appraisal Processing." *Journal of Abnormal Child Psychology* 37 (7): 945–56. https://doi.org/10.1007/s10802-009-9321-5.

Flook, Lisa, Simon B. Goldberg, Laura Pinger, Katherine Bonus, and Richard J. Davidson. 2013. "Mindfulness for Teachers: A Pilot Study to Assess Effects on Stress, Burnout, and Teaching Efficacy." *Mind, Brain, and Education* 7 (3): 182–95.

Fogel, Alan. 1993. *Developing through Relationships: Origins of Communication, Self, and Culture.* Chicago: University of Chicago Press.

Granata, Kassondra. 2020. "10 Social Justice Ideas to Try in Class." *Education World.* Accessed March 19, 2021. https://www.educationworld.com/a_lesson/social-justice-activities-students.shtml.

Greater Good Science Center. n.d. "What Is Mindfulness?" Accessed May 11, 2021. https://greatergood.berkeley.edu/topic/mindfulness/definition#why-practice.

Hamilton, David R. 2011. "5 Beneficial Side Effects of Kindness." *HuffPost*, August 2, 2011. https://www.huffpost.com/entry/kindness-benefits_b_869537.

Hareli, Shlomo, and Ursula Hess. 2010. "What Emotional Reactions Can Tell Us about the Nature of Others: An Appraisal Perspective on Person Perception." *Cognition and Emotion* 24 (1): 128–40. https://doi.org/10.1080/02699930802613828.

Harpin, Scott B., AnneMarie Rossi, Amber K. Kim, and Leah M. Swanson. 2016. "Behavioral Impacts of a Mindfulness Pilot Intervention for Elementary School Students." *Education* 137 (2): 149–56.

International Dyslexia Association. 2018. "Scarborough's Reading Rope: A Groundbreaking Infographic." *International Dyslexia Association (IDA)* 7 (2). https://dyslexiaida.org/scarboroughs-reading-rope-a-groundbreaking-infographic/.

Jennings, Patricia A., and Mark T. Greenberg. 2009. "The Prosocial Classroom: Teacher Social and Emotional Competence in Relation to Student and Classroom Outcomes." *Review of Educational Research* 79 (1): 491–525.

Jones, Damon E., Mark Greenberg, and Max Crowley. 2015. "Early Social-Emotional Functioning and Public Health: The Relationship between Kindergarten Social Competence and Future Wellness." *American Journal of Public Health* 105 (11): 2283–90.

Kagan, Spencer. 1994. *Cooperative Learning.* San Clemente, CA: Resources for Teachers, Inc.

Kern, Margaret L., Howard S. Friedman, Leslie R. Martin, Chandra A. Reynolds, and Gloria Luong. 2009. "Conscientiousness, Career Success, and Longevity: A Lifespan Analysis." *Annals of Behavioral Medicine* 37 (2): 154–63. https://doi.org/10.1007/s12160-009-9095-6.

Kidd, Celeste, Holly Palmeri, and Richard N. Aslin. 2013. "Rational Snacking: Young Children's Decision-Making on the Marshmallow Task Is Moderated by Beliefs about Environmental Reliability." *Cognition* 126 (1): 109–14. https://doi.org/10.1016/j.cognition.2012.08.004.

Knudsen, Eric I., James J. Heckman, Judy L. Cameron, and Jack P. Shonkoff. 2006. "Economic, Neurobiological, and Behavioral Perspectives on Building America's Future Workforce." *Proceedings of the National Academy of Sciences* 103 (27): 10155–62.

Layous, Kristin, S. Katherine Nelson, Eva Oberle, Kimberly A. Schonert-Reichl, and Sonja Lyubomirsky. 2012. "Kindness Counts: Prompting Prosocial Behavior in Preadolescents Boosts Peer Acceptance and Well-Being." *PLoS One* 7 (12). https://www.ncbi.nlm.nih.gov /pmc/articles/PMC3530573/.

Manstead, Antony S. R. 2018. "The Psychology of Social Class: How Socioeconomic Status Impacts Thought, Feelings, and Behavior." *British Journal of Social Psychology* 57: 267–91. https://doi.org/10.1111/bjso.12251.

Martel, Michelle M., Joel T. Nigg, Maria M. Wong, Hiram E. Fitzgerald, Jennifer M. Jester, Leon I. Puttler, Jennifer M. Glass, Kenneth M. Adams, and Robert A. Zucker. 2007. "Childhood and Adolescent Resiliency, Regulation, and Executive Functioning in Relation to Adolescent Problems and Competence in a High-Risk Sample." *Development and Psychopathology* 19 (2): 541–63. https://doi.org/10.1017/S0954579407070265.

McClelland, Megan M., Claire E. Cameron, Shannon B. Wanless, and Amy Murray. 2007. "Executive Function, Behavioral Self-Regulation, and Social-Emotional Competence: Links to School Readiness." In *Contemporary Perspectives on Social Learning in Early Childhood Education*, edited by Olivia N. Saracho and Bernard Spodek, 83–107. Charlotte, NC: Information Age Publishing.

Mitchem, Katherine J., K. Richard Young, Richard P. West, and Julieann Benyo. 2001. "CWPASM: A Classwide Peer-Assisted Self-Management Program for General Education Classrooms." *Education and Treatment of Children* 24 (2): 111–40.

Moffitt, Terrie E., Louise Arseneault, Daniel Belsky, Nigel Dickson, Robert J. Hancox, HonaLee Harrington, Renate Houts, et al. 2011. "A Gradient of Childhood Self-Control Predicts Health, Wealth, and Public Safety." *Proceedings of the National Academy of Sciences* 108 (7): 2693–98. https://doi.org/10.1073/pnas.1010076108.

Moos, Daniel C., and Alyssa Ringdal. 2012. "Self-Regulated Learning in the Classroom: A Literature Review on the Teacher's Role." *Education Research International* 2012. https://www.hindawi.com/journals/edri/2012/423284/.

National Institute of Mental Health. n.d. "Suicide Is a Leading Cause of Death in the United States." Accessed May 11, 2021. https://www.nimh.nih.gov/health/statistics/suicide .shtml.

O'Connor, Erin E., Eric Dearing, Brian A. Collins. 2011. "Teacher-Child Relationship and Behavior Problem Trajectories in Elementary School." *American Educational Research Journal* 48 (1): 120–62.

Oettingen, Gabriele. 2015. *Rethinking Positive Thinking: Inside the New Science of Motivation.* New York: Current.

Okun, Michael S., Dawn Bowers, Utaka Springer, Nathan A. Shapira, Donald Malone, Ali R. Rezai, Bart Nuttin, et al. 2004. "What's in a 'Smile'? Intra-Operative Observations of Contralateral Smiles Induced by Deep Brain Stimulation." *Neurocase* 10 (4): 271–79. https://doi.org/10.1080/13554790490507632.

Parkinson, Brian. 2001. "Putting Appraisal in Context." In *Appraisal Processes in Emotion: Theory, Methods, Research,* edited by Klaus R. Scherer, Angela Schorr, and Tom Johnstone, 173–86. Oxford, UK: Oxford University Press.

Parkinson, Brian, and Sarah Illingworth. 2009. "Guilt in Response to Blame from Others." *Cognition & Emotion* 23 (8): 1589–1614.

Perou, Ruth, Rebecca H. Bitsko, Stephen J. Blumberg, Patricia Pastor, Reem M. Ghandour, and Joseph C. Gfroerer et al. 2013. "Mental Health Surveillance Among Children—United States, 2005–2011." *Morbidity and Mortality Weekly Report (MMWR)*, May 17, 2013. www.cdc.gov/mmwr/preview/mmwrhtml/su6202a1.htm?s_cid=su6202a1_w.

Raaijmakers, Maartje A., Diana P. Smidts, Joseph A. Sergeant, Gerard H. Maassen, Jocelyne A. Posthumus, Herman van Engeland, and Walter Matthys. 2008. "Executive Functions in Preschool Children with Aggressive Behavior: Impairments in Inhibitory Control." *Journal of Abnormal Child Psychology* 36: 1097–1107. https://doi.org/10.1007/s10802-008-9235-7.

Segal, Zindel V., Peter Bieling, Trevor Young, Glenda MacQueen, Robert Cooke, Lawrence Martin, Richard Bloch, and Robert D. Levitan. 2010. "Antidepressant Monotherapy vs Sequential Pharmacotherapy and Mindfulness-Based Cognitive Therapy, or Placebo, for Relapse Prophylaxis in Recurrent Depression." *Archives of General Psychiatry* 67 (12): 1256–64. https://doi.org/10.1001/archgenpsychiatry.2010.168.

Sesame Workshop. 2016. "K Is for Kind: A National Survey on Kindness and Kids." http://kindness.sesamestreet.org/view-the-results/.

Siegel, Daniel J. 2010. *Mindsight: The New Science of Personal Transformation.* New York: Bantam.

Silver, Rebecca B., Jeffrey R. Measelle, Jeffrey M. Armstrong, and Marilyn J. Essex. 2005. "Trajectories of Classroom Externalizing Behavior: Contributions of Child Characteristics, Family Characteristics, and the Teacher-Child Relationship During the School Transition." *Journal of School Psychology* 43 (1): 39–60.

Simmons, Dena. 2019. "Why We Can't Afford Whitewashed Social-Emotional Learning." *ASCD Education Update* 61 (4): (April). http://www.ascd.org/publications/newsletters/education_update/apr19/vol61/num04/Why_We_Can't_Afford_Whitewashed_Social-Emotional_Learning.aspx.

Sutin, Angelina R., Luigi Ferrucci, Alan B. Zonderman, and Antonio Terracciano. 2011. "Personality and Obesity across the Adult Life Span." *Journal of Personality and Social Psychology* 101 (3): 579–92. https://doi.org/10.1037/a0024286.

Tarullo, Amanda R., Jelena Obradović, and Megan R. Gunnar. 2009. "Self-Control and the Developing Brain." *Zero to Three* 29 (3): 31–37.

Taylor, Rebecca D., Eva Oberle, Joseph A. Durlak, and Roger P. Weissburg. 2017. "Promoting Positive Youth Development through School-Based Social and Emotional Learning Interventions: A Meta-Analysis of Follow-Up Effects." *Child Development* 88 (4): 1156–71.

University of Toronto. 2010. "Inner Voice Plays Role in Self Control." *ScienceDaily*, September 22, 2010. https://www.sciencedaily.com/releases/2010/09/100921110956.htm.

Wang, Margaret C., Geneva D. Haertel, and Herbert J. Walberg. 1990. "What Influences Learning? A Content Analysis of Review Literature." *The Journal of Educational Research* 84 (1): 30–43.

Williams, Amanda, Kelly O'Driscoll, and Chris Moore. 2014. "The Influence of Empathic Concern on Prosocial Behavior in Children." *Frontiers in Psychology* 5: 425. https://doi.org/10.3389/fpsyg.2014.00425.

Wright, Jim. n.d. "Self-Check Behavior Checklist Maker." *Intervention Central.* Accessed March 30, 2021. https://www.interventioncentral.org/tools/self-check-behavior-checklist-maker.

Digital Resources

Accessing the Digital Resources

The Digital Resources can be downloaded by following these steps:

1. Go to **www.tcmpub.com/digital**

2. Use the ISBN number to redeem the Digital Resources.

> **ISBN: 978-1-0876-4885-9**

3. Respond to the question using the book.

4. Follow the prompts on the Content Cloud website to sign in or create a new account.

5. Choose the Digital Resources you would like to download. You can download all the files at once, or a specific group of files.

   ▸ **Please note:** Some files provided for download have large file sizes. Download times for these larger files vary based on your download speed.